MAN'S WORLD *digest*

No.5, being a digest of MAN'S WORLD Issue 12 / Fall 2023

MAN'S WORLD

digest #5

CONTENTS

MAN'S WORLD

RAW EGG NATIONALIST

editor-in-chief

RAW EGG NATIONALIST

editorial director

RAW EGG NATIONALIST

deputy editor

RAW EGG NATIONALIST

art director

RAW EGG NATIONALIST

deputy editor's assistant

RAW EGG NATIONALIST   *editor at large*

EDITORIAL

COPY: RAW EGG NATIONALIST

RESEARCH: RAW EGG NATIONALIST

STAFF: RAW EGG NATIONALIST

ART

RAW EGG NATIONALIST

senior art director

RAW EGG NATIONALIST

art coordinator

PUBLIC RELATIONS

RAW EGG NATIONALIST

vice president / director

ADVERTISING

GLOBAL: RAW EGG NATIONALIST

"EDITORIAL HARASSMENT!"

Welcome back, MAN'S WORLD fans! First of all, let me thank you again, from the bottom of my black little heart, for buying this, the fifth edition of the MAN'S WORLD Digest, and helping to support the work I do. This entire enterprise lives — and hopefully never dies — on the basis of you being kind enough to read and share the articles on the site, retweet our posts on Twitter (follow @mansworldmag_) and occasionally shell out on a Digest, Annual or one of our fantastic new t-shirts, available from the MAN'S WORLD Store.

On the subject of t-shirts, we have some fantastic designs you can wear to show your support for the embattled 45th President of the United States. Whatever your opinions about the man, it's clear that the United States has reached a true inflection point in its history. The fate of the Republic hangs in the balance, and Trump is the central character in this drama. Nobody else in the Republican party matters at this point. I know, as much as anybody else, the faults and failures of the man and his first term as president, but nothing changes the fact that, if his opponents succeed and jail him or prevent him from winning the election, the chances of any kind of American revival are pretty much slim to none.

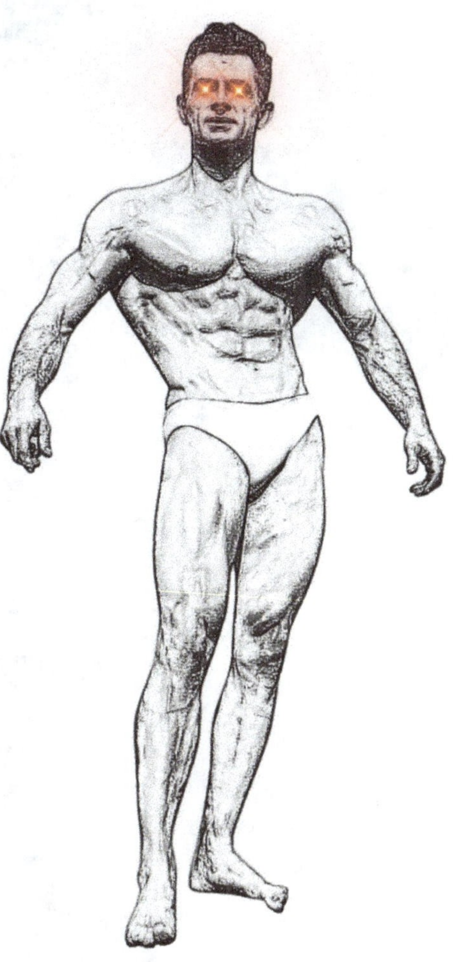

@babygravy9

Anyway, we've got a fantastic Digest, maybe the best Digest yet, so you're in for a real treat. Two essays by me, including a scorching Counterblast polemic against any and all entryists who think internet anonymity is just a vehicle for their own personal ambition. Stable genius SCOTT GREER has a great piece on Andrew Tate, and we also have essays on Yukio Mishima, the Conquistadors, the battle over America's sacred history and much more.

Oh end before I sign off, we've got a huge announcemnt coming in the new year: so what this space!

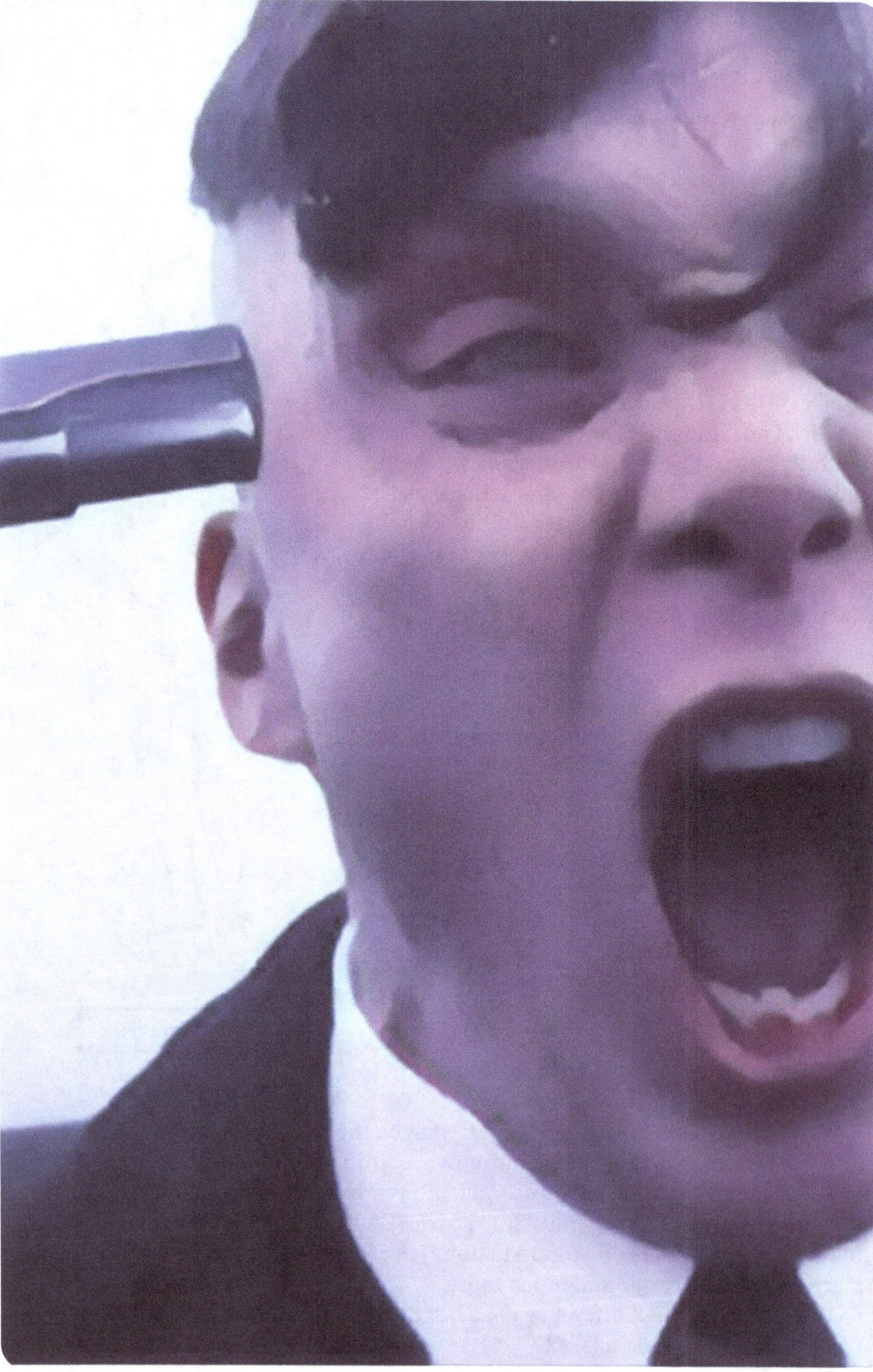

IT'S OVER (WE'RE SO BACK)

essay by RAW EGG NATIONALIST

Take courage: there are plenty of things we can do to protect ourselves against the estrogenic and obesogenic chemicals that are poisoning our world...

It was a Saturday afternoon, if I recall correctly, and I had been browsing PubMed as I so often do, covfefe in hand, looking for brand new studies to write about. I usually search by simple terms – "testosterone", "microplastics", "PFAS", "soy manboobs" ("soy gynecomastia", to use the technical term) and so on. On this occasion, it was "endocrine disruptors", which, if you don't know, are chemicals that interfere with the body's natural hormonal balance.

I scrolled down the page, scanning each entry listed in chronological order. Not much. And then I saw it: "Can oestrogenic activity in air contribute to the overall body burden of endocrine disruptors?", in the journal *Environmental Toxicology and Pharmacology*.

Could it really be, I asked myself: is the air feminising us!? Can breathing literally make us less masculine!? I didn't doubt it. It's 2023, after all, and literally everything is gay. The food is gay. The water is gay. The culture is gay. So why not the air too?

I read the abstract with some excitement and then the full paper and, yes, it would appear that the air is contributing "to the overall body burden of endocrine disruptors" – which means, in short, that the air *is* feminising us.

Here's what the study involved. Researchers in Italy took samples of particulate matter from the air in five different locations in the north of the country (an area of busy traffic, an urban area, a site near an incinerator and two separate rural spots). Samples were taken in all four seasons at each location. The researchers then measured each sample for cytotoxicity (toxicity to living cells) and estrogenicity (activity mimicking the effects of the hormone estrogen). The estrogenicity test was performed with the drug tamoxifen, a selective estrogen receptor modulator that's used primarily to prevent breast cancer.

What the researchers found was that all of the samples exhibited significant estrogenic activity, in addition to heavy cytotoxicity. Chemicals of interest were benzo(a)pyrene and also pesticides, bisphenol A, alkylphenols, polybrominated diphenyl ethers, polychlorinated biphenyls and polychlorinated dibenzodioxins or dibenzofurans. These chemicals have nasty names for good reason.

Notably, there was a clear seasonal variation at all sites, with the autumn and winter samples showing the most estrogenic activity. This can be explained by the fact that, at lower temperatures, the chemicals identified are more likely to sit in the air as particulate rather than existing in a gaseous state, meaning there was more of them in the samples.

I found it particularly interesting that, although one of the rural areas had, as we might expect, the best air, exhibiting the lowest cytotoxicity and estrogenicity, the other had worse air quality than the incinerator site, and was barely superior to the air from the traffic and urban locations. If there was some particular reason for this, the researchers didn't say, but it could easily have been because of nearby agricultural activity – crop spraying, etc – or even the burning of tires, which is more and more of a pastime the further south and east you go in Europe.

Needless to say, logging on to the bird app, I knew I was on to a winner. "IT'S OFFICIALLY OVER", I titled the thread, and accompanied it with a picture of doomer wojak in Bosch's Hell. I described the method and the results of the study in detail and then ended with the suggestion that it might be time we all started "Bane-maxxing" to protect our gains, i.e. wearing masks. This was not a serious suggestion. But I should have known better. Because if there's anything the average Twitter user is renowned for, it isn't understanding how to read basic verbal and contextual cues.

The post had millions of views and, ominously, thousands of quote tweets and replies. Calling out from among the bemused comments that I was advocating a return to masking a la COVID-19 ("right wingers are now mask cucks") or that I was displaying a "feminisation fetish" (I secretly want to be made a sissy by the air?), I heard a refrain that I could actually understand: If everything, even the air, is toxic, what's the point in caring? What can we actually do about it?

The next day I wrote a response thread, hoping to clarify my intentions about the post and about my posts in general on the subject. I want to pick up on what I said there and say it again, because I think it needs repeating.

Yes, it's easy to become overwhelmed by the sheer scale of the problem of environmental pollution and its effects on human health and

"IT'S 2023 AND LITERALLY EVERYTHING IS GAY. THE FOOD IS GAY. THE WATER IS GAY. THE CULTURE IS GAY. SO WHY NOT THE AIR TOO?"

fertility. Barely a day passes without multiple new studies on pollutants and substances like microplastics or some fresh Jeremiad about the future of the human race. The most headline-grabbing prediction has been Professor Shanna Swan's claim that by 2045, mankind as a species may be unable to reproduce by natural means. This is just an extrapolation of current trends. If declines in sperm counts continue at the same rate, in a little over twenty years the median man will have a sperm count of zero: one half of all men will produce no sperm, and the other half will produce so few that they might as well produce none. This is often referred to as "spermageddon".

There are many ways a person could react to this problem on social media. One way would be just to point to the problem and say, "it's over". And before you say, "That's exactly what you did!", let me reiterate that the tweet was intended to be strictly tongue in cheek. If you've seen my other tweets or read my essays in *American Mind, American Greatness*, the *Epoch Times* or anywhere else, or indeed if you've read my book *The Eggs Benedict Option*, you'll know that I've always done my best to make clear that what we need is not more despair, but a determined political solution, a movement to reclaim our health and wellbeing and rejuvenate our nations.

We can already see the beginnings of such a movement with Robert F. Kennedy Jr., who is making the health of America a political issue in a way it probably hasn't been – ever. Yes, there have been health crusades, such as Nixon's War on Cancer, but the focus was only ever on individual conditions, not health in general. Whether Kennedy is the right candidate isn't clear at this point, but he's already had a salutary effect on the terms of this election cycle. In a clear response to Kennedy's bid for the presidency, Donald Trump announced that he would launch a presidential commission into chronic diseases, to investigate the root causes of American's unprecedented ill health. This isn't something I could imagine Trump doing otherwise.

Such a movement won't emerge overnight, and any positive changes that are made will take years, maybe decades, to have their full effect. In the meantime, there are plenty of things we can do in our daily lives to begin reclaiming our health as individuals, and I've always gone out of my way to try to tell you what they are. Small interventions can make a huge difference. It's well known, for example, that women's exposure to endocrine-disrupting chemicals is massively increased through use of personal-care and beauty products.

A study of college-age girls showed that, on average, they use eight personal-care and beauty products a day that contain endocrine-disrupting chemicals, with some of the girls in the sample using as many as 17. It's not a wonder, then, that simply not using these products is one of the best things girls and women can do to protect their health. Doing just that, as another study showed, can reduce levels of chemicals like bisphenol A and phthalates in girls' urine by as much as 45%.

Filter your water. Stop eating processed food and choose organic local produce instead. Ditch as much plastic as you can. Exercise and get plenty of sunlight. These things are more than enough to make your life immeasurably better, in a surprisingly short period of time. Not one of them will mark you out as a weirdo – well, not much of a weirdo – or in any way compromise your quality of life.

We can't totally avoid exposure to harmful industrial chemicals, but we can reduce our exposure to them and do simple things that counteract their effects, at the same time as pushing for political change that will rid our environment of these substances – maybe one day for good. There is no reason to abandon hope. So whatever the doomers may tell you, it's not over. Actually, you could even say *we're so back.* ◼

THE MORALIST

Was I Right To Call the Guards on a Western Steppe Herder Stealing My Daughter?

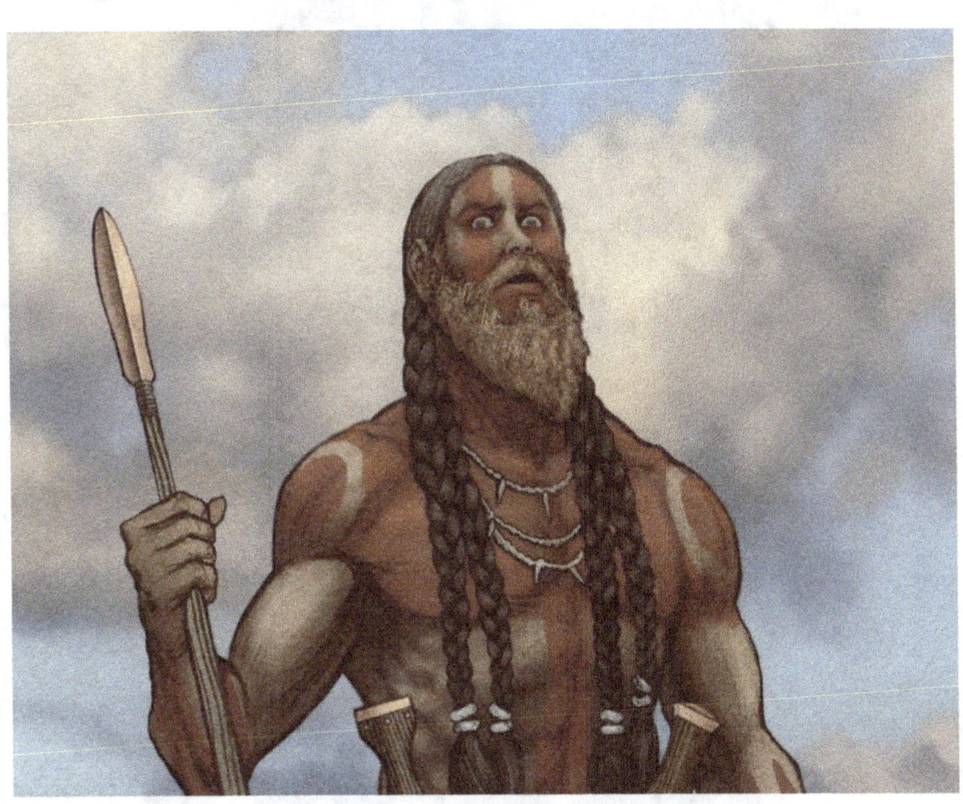

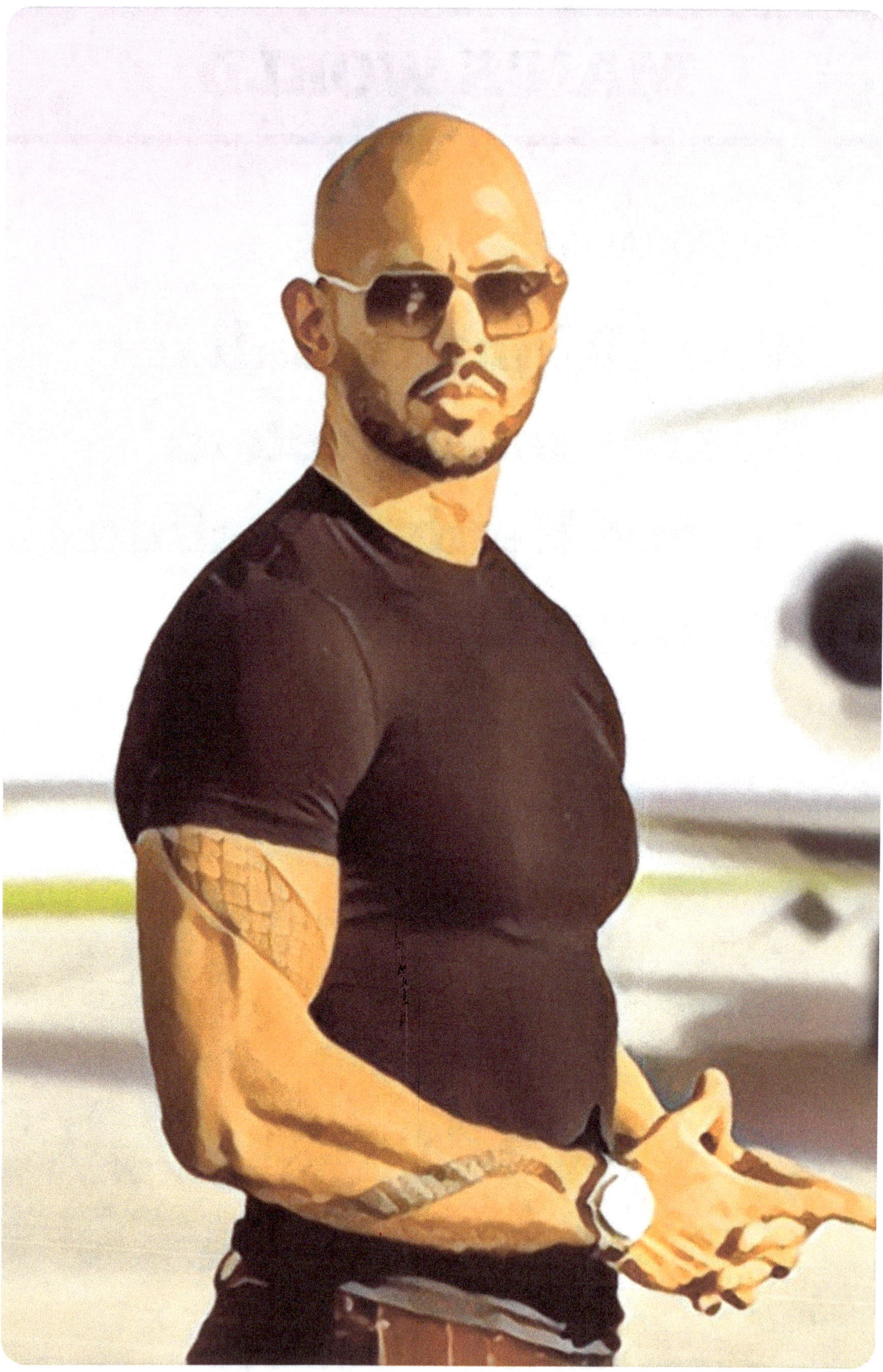

THE HERO AMERICA DESERVES

essay by SCOTT GREER

As much as conservative proponents of Good Masculinity may say otherwise, Andrew Tate is exactly the kind of man who best represents their movement...

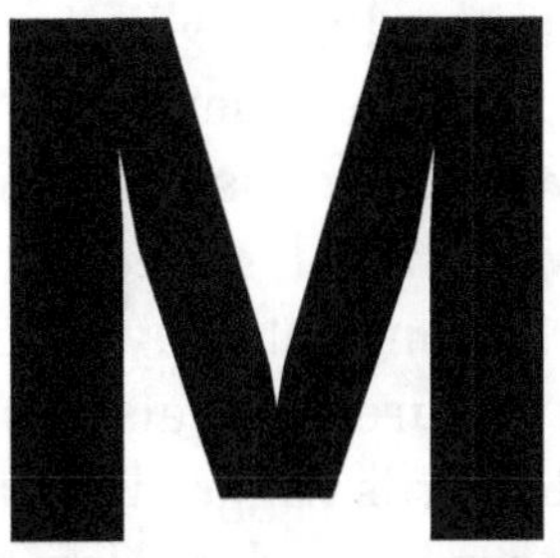

Most conservative movement activists hate Andrew Tate with a burning passion. In their eyes, Tate is no more than a sexist pimp. He's a bad influence on young men. He's not a "real man" because he doesn't encourage his followers to get married, have children, and vote for GOP candidates. In short, Andrew Tate is not a True Conservative.

Conservative pundits fixated on the "Crisis of Masculinity" use Tate as an example of what *leftism* produces. Josh Hawley, for example, says Tate is "a child pretending to be a man" because he tells men that women like to be choked during sex. Sexual asphyxiation must be a major cause of the GOOD MEN shortage!

The irony, of course, is that Andrew Tate embodies the multi-racial working class movement that Hawley and his ilk promote so desperately. Tate's massive audience includes lower status ethnic groups (the former kickboxer is mixed-race himself). His hustler ethos has more appeal among working class men than any DC meme ideology. If multiracial working class conservatism were real, Tate would be its leader.

Tate's philosophy is a more polished variant of the rap ethos "Fuck Bitches, Get Money." He exudes over-the-top machismo, finds self-worth in ostentatious displays of wealth, and emphasizes a gang mentality among friends. But Tate takes the rap lifestyle out of the ghetto. His appeal is not black-coded: it's open to all. Though he sometimes speaks the language of criminals, Tate doesn't want his audience to become gangbangers. He promises to make them middle-class entrepreneurs, sans the old bourgeois values and norms. He raises rap values to a level that can appeal equally to white suburbanites and working-class minorities.

In some ways, Tate's "hustler" mentality is a cynical and classless variant of the American Dream. Both emphasize hard work (called the "grindset" in Tate's world), dedication, prosperity, and the entrepreneurial spirit. Hustlers University promises to turn its "students" into rich capitalists. One could say Tate is a Horatio Alger for the 21st century.

The differences between Tate and past exponents of the American Dream are obvious. He ridicules middle class careerists as "brokies" and doesn't pay much lip service to family men. He promotes a life of extravagant opulence rather than middling comfort. Tate is not a Christian and, despite his newfound Islamic faith, dispenses with social conservatism. He encourages his followers to become rich and successful men more than good husbands.

Everything about Tate's style is an affront to WASP taste. He doesn't sport Brooks Brothers and loafers. He encourages more discrete bling than rappers, but still flaunts bedazzled watches and expensive sports cars. Tate's celebration of excessive spending and gaudiness flies in the face of WASP thrift and

inconspicuousness. His semi-gangster machismo would be frowned upon at a country club. WASPs hardly know what a Bugatti is, let alone brag about owning one.

Andrew Tate's American Dream will represent the right in a post-White America. The traditional WASP values associated with conservatism and the Republican Party will die out with the Baby Boomer generation. Young whites today have zero aspiration to reproduce the WASP ideal, raised as they were in a world dominated by rap music and black culture. They also don't want to sink towards wiggerdom, a direction many are headed in. Non-whites don't want to be WASPs either, but they fear getting stuck in the ghetto. And neither group enjoys the constant lectures from prissy, moralistic liberal women. Tate offers something different from WASP-dom and the ghetto lifestyle. He promotes a lavish, male fantasy.

Andrew Tate's hustler ethos appeals to both white Americans who want to shed their whiteness and non-whites who want to achieve material prosperity. His transgressive male sensibility speaks to young men bashed over the head with feminine moralism (from both right and left) their entire lives. They want to make money and fuck beautiful women. And while most Tate adherents will not drive sports cars or hang out on yachts, they may rationalize their middle class striving as a

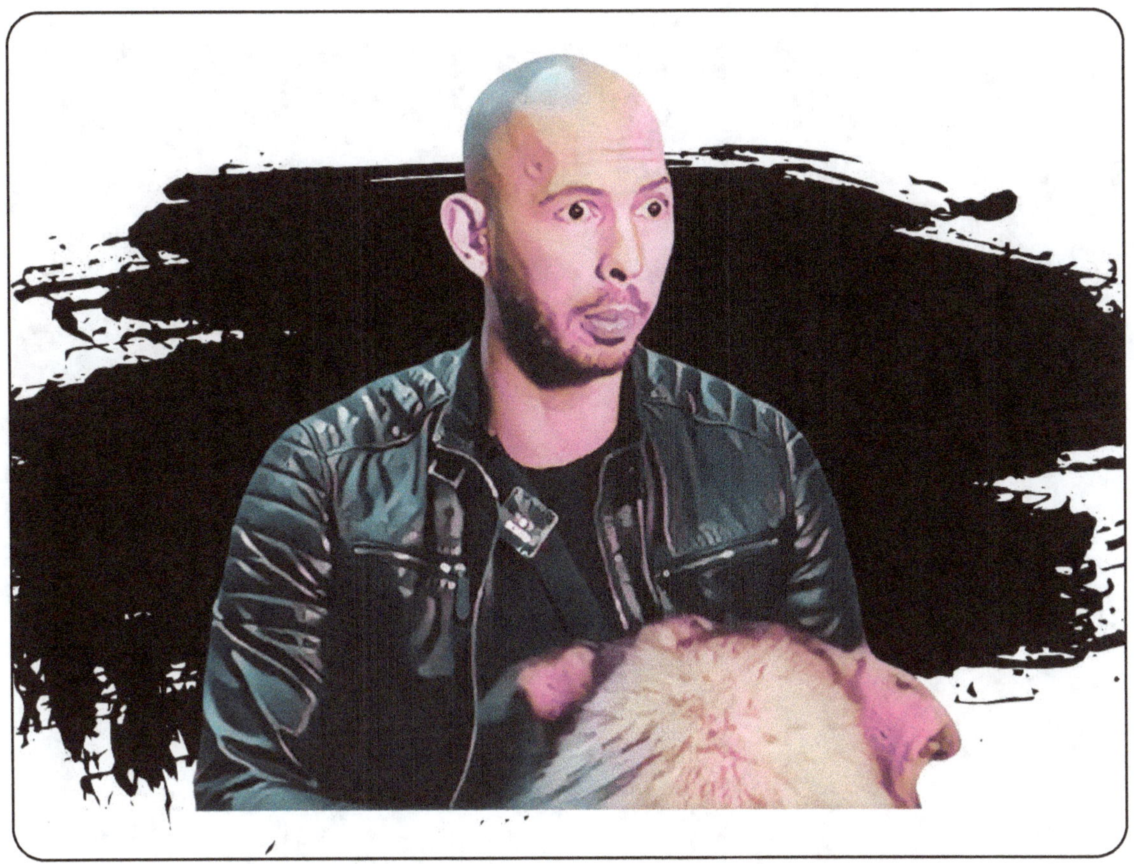

Tate-style hustle. It's just a new "self-help" guide for such men to reach the suburban ideal. Hustlerism has a much broader appeal in a majority-white nation beset with anti-white racism.

Postliberals who loathe Tate imagine the multiracial working class as resolutely anti-capitalist. Anyone familiar with "grindset" knows blacks and Hispanics don't want to overthrow the capitalist system. They want to game it to achieve the American Dream. This, of course, often leads them into pyramid schemes and other harebrained endeavors – which Tate seems to actively promote. But their stupid attempts don't disabuse them of American capitalism. The promise of wealth attracts them more than the pseudo-Marxism espoused by an irrelevant Beltway intelligentsia.

Conservatives and postliberals insist the multiracial working class is socially conservative. There's some truth to that, but not in the sense you'd find in the pages of a conservative magazine. Young men who watch Tate videos are not avid churchgoers waiting for marriage. The majority of them never go to church. They don't want to live in a society run by clerics. They just dislike the excesses of wokeness and feminism. Tate, as stated above, is no social conservative. He makes his money off OnlyFans girls and encourages sexual promiscuity. At the same time, he attacks feminism and political correctness. Conservatives may scoff, but this reflects the beliefs of young American men far more than any integralist.

This is not to praise Hustlerism. It would be much better for young Americans to aspire to WASP etiquette and decorum. Andrew Tate wouldn't be

FILTERED CRAFT CIGARETTES
HESTIA

NAKED, WILD,
TOBACCO.

Hestia supports rich soil, healthy plants, and absolutely delicious tobacco. Our farmers grow naked, unadulterated tobacco as it was grown long before governments codified "organic." To give you the finest, our farmers are free to grow the healthiest and best possible tobacco, what many have done for over eight generations, tending their wild land and naked plants, ensuring their soil is happy and dynamic, guaranteeing your cigarettes are the very best.

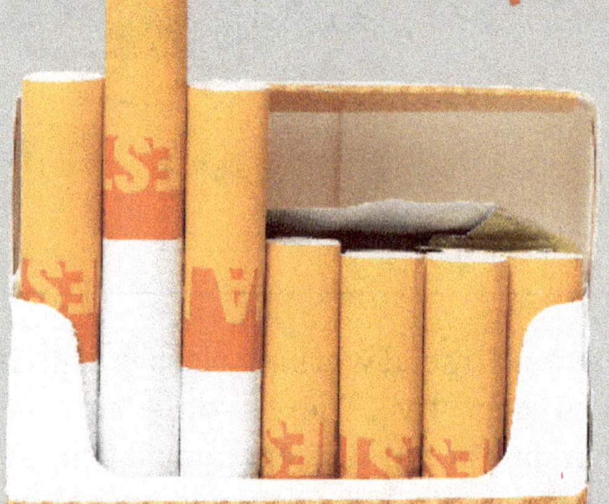
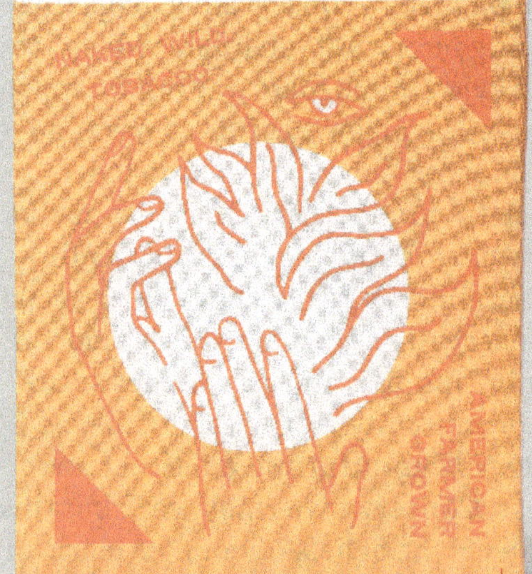

NAKED WILD
TOBACCO
AMERICAN FARMER GROWN

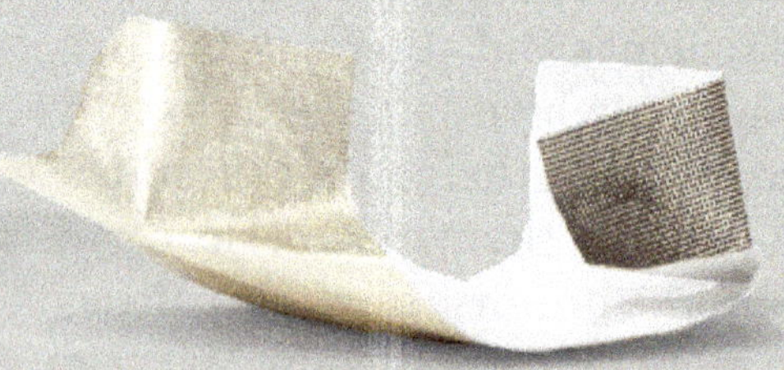

HESTIATOBACCO.COM

@HESTIATOBACCO

SURGEON GENERAL'S WARNING: CIGARETTE SMOKE CONTAINS CARBON MONOXIDE.

popular in a whiter country. But we are moving towards a post-white America, and Tate's politics and self-presentation will only become more common. Conservatism in a majority-minority America looks like the former kickboxer, minus his recent conversion to Islam. It will be secular, diverse, hyper-capitalist, and anti-woke. It will not care about gay marriage or abortion. It will not dress in polos and khakis. It will not desire the Empire of Our Lady of Guadalupe.

In practice, multiracial working class conservatism will want a new version of the American Dream – complete with rap music and gold chains. It will want Andrew Tate. ◾

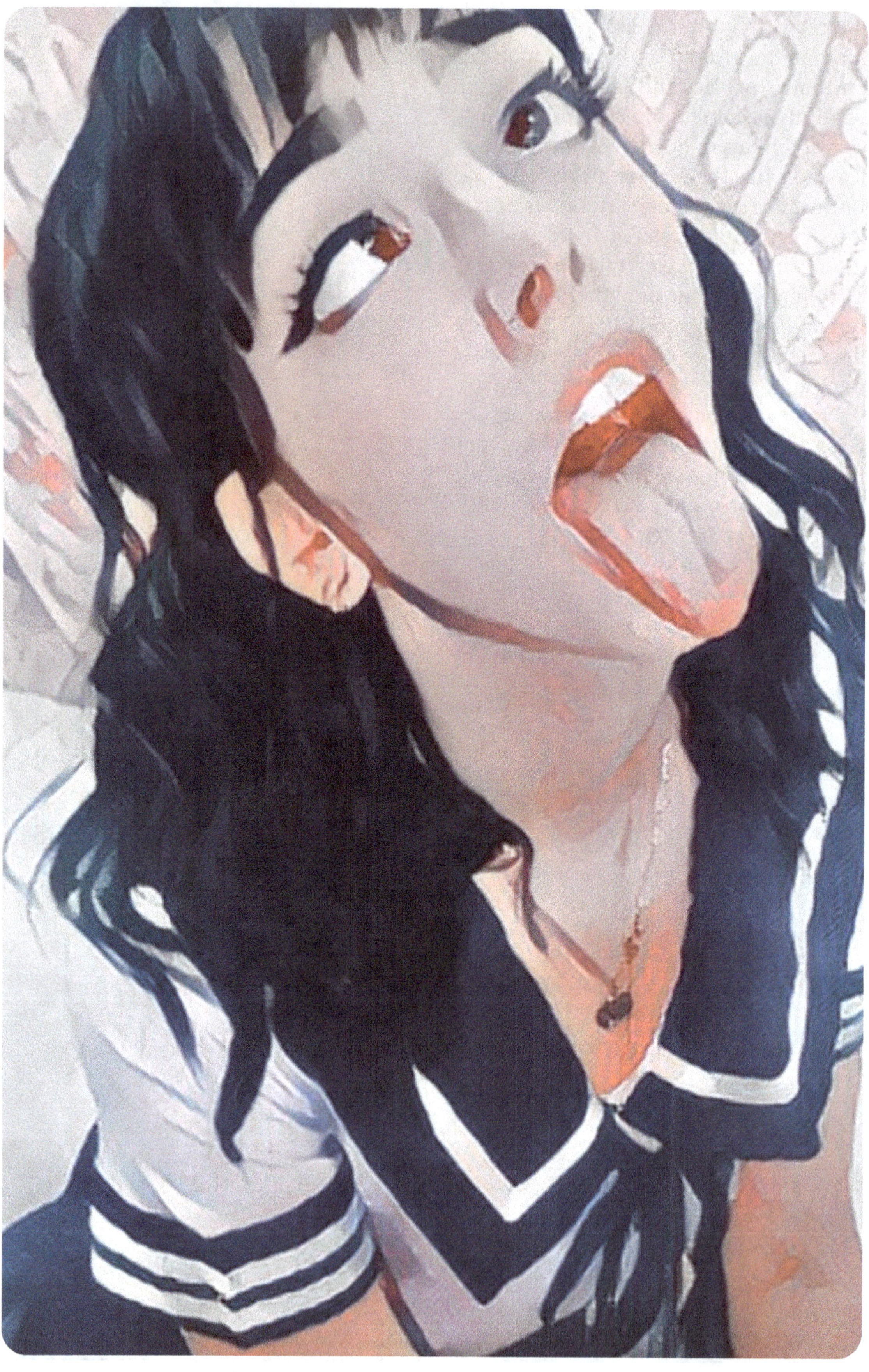

ON WOMEN

classic essay by ARTHUR SCHOPENHAUER

*The great philosopher's classic essay on the so-called
"fairer sex", which has generated plenty of controversy on
Twitter thanks to a certain Bronze Age Pervert...*

These few words of Jouy, *Sans les femmes le commence-
ment de notre vie seroit privé de secours, le milieu de plaisirs
et la fin de consolation* ["Without women, the beginning
of our life would be helpless; the middle, devoid of
pleasure; and the end, of consolation"), more exactly
express, in my opinion, the true praise of woman than Schiller's
poem, *Würde der Frauen*, which is the fruit of much careful thought
and impressive because of its antithesis and use of contrast. The
same thing is more pathetically expressed by Byron in *Sardanapalus*,
Act i, Sc. 2:—

> "The very first
> Of human life must spring from woman's breast,
> Your first small words are taught you from her lips,
> Your first tears quench'd by her, and your last sighs
> Too often breathed out in a woman's hearing,
> When men have shrunk from the ignoble care
> Of watching the last hour of him who led them."

Both passages show the right point of view for the appreciation
of women.

One need only look at a woman's shape to discover that she is
not intended for either too much mental or too much physical work.
She pays the debt of life not by what she does but by what she suffers—by the pains of child-bearing, care for the child, and by sub-

jection to man, to whom she should be a patient and cheerful companion. The greatest sorrows and joys or great exhibition of strength are not assigned to her; her life should flow more quietly, more gently, and less obtrusively than man's, without her being essentially happier or unhappier.

Women are directly adapted to act as the nurses and educators of our early childhood, for the simple reason that they themselves are childish, foolish, and short-sighted—in a word, are big children all their lives, something intermediate between the child and the man, who is a man in the strict sense of the word. Consider how a young girl will toy day after day with a child, dance with it and sing to it; and then consider what a man, with the very best intentions in the world, could do in her place.

With girls, Nature has had in view what is called in a dramatic sense a "striking effect," for she endows them for a few years with a richness of beauty and a, fulness of charm at the expense of the rest of their lives; so that they may during these years ensnare the fantasy of a man to such a degree as to make him rush into taking the honourable care of them, in some kind of form, for a lifetime—a step which would not seem sufficiently justified if he only considered the matter. Accordingly, Nature has furnished woman, as she has the rest of her creatures, with the weapons and implements necessary for the protection of her existence and for just the length of time that they will be of service to her; so that Nature has proceeded here with her usual economy. Just as the female ant after coition loses her wings, which then become superfluous, nay, dangerous for breeding purposes, so for the most part does a woman lose her beauty after giving birth to one or two children; and probably for the same reasons.

Then again we find that young girls in their hearts regard their domestic or other affairs as secondary things, if not as a mere jest. Love, conquests, and all that these include, such as dressing, dancing, and so on, they give their serious attention.

The nobler and more perfect a thing is, the later and slower is it in reaching maturity. Man reaches the maturity of his reasoning and mental faculties scarcely before he is eight-and-twenty; woman when she is eighteen; but hers is reason of very narrow limitations. This is why women remain children all their lives, for they always see only what is near at hand, cling to the present, take the appearance of a thing for reality, and prefer trifling matters to the most important. It is by virtue of man's reasoning powers that he does not live in the present only, like the brute, but observes and ponders over the past and future; and from this spring discretion, care, and that anxiety which we so frequently notice in people. The advantages, as well as the disadvantages, that this entails, make woman, in consequence of her weaker reasoning powers, less of a partaker in them. Moreover, she is intellectually short-sighted, for although her intuitive understanding quickly perceives what is near to her, on the other hand her circle of vision is limited and does not embrace anything that is remote; hence everything that is absent or past, or in the future, affects women in a less degree than men. This is why they have greater inclination for extravagance, which sometimes borders on madness.

"NATURE HAS MADE IT THE CALLING OF THE YOUNG, STRONG, AND HANDSOME MEN TO LOOK AFTER THE PROPAGATION OF THE HUMAN RACE"

Women in their hearts think that men are intended to earn money so that they may spend it, if possible during their husband's lifetime, but at any rate after his death.

As soon as he has given them his earnings on which to keep house they are strengthened in this belief. Although all this entails many disadvantages, yet it has this advantage—that a woman lives more in the present than a man, and that she enjoys it more keenly if it is at all bearable. This is the origin of that cheerfulness which is peculiar to woman and makes her fit to divert man, and in case of need, to console him when he is weighed down by cares. To consult women in matters of difficulty, as the Germans used to do in old times, is by no means a matter to be overlooked; for their way of grasping a thing is quite different from ours, chiefly because they like the shortest way to the point, and usually keep their attention fixed upon what lies nearest; while we, as a rule, see beyond it, for the simple reason that it lies under our nose; it then becomes necessary for us to be brought back to the thing in order to obtain a near and simple view. This is why women are more sober in their judgment than we, and why they see nothing more in things than is really there; while we, if our passions are roused, slightly exaggerate or add to our imagination.

It is because women's reasoning powers are weaker that they show more sympathy for the unfortunate than men, and consequently take a kindlier interest in them. On the other hand, women are inferior to men in matters of justice, honesty, and conscientiousness. Again, because their reasoning faculty is weak, things clearly visible and real, and belonging to the present, exercise a power over them which is rarely counteracted by abstract thoughts, fixed maxims, or firm resolutions, in general, by regard for the past and future or by consideration for what is absent and remote. Accordingly they have the first and principal qualities of virtue, but they lack the secondary qualities which are often a necessary instrument in developing it. Women may be compared in this respect to an organism that has a liver but no gall-bladder. So that it will be found that the fundamental fault in the character of women is that they have no *sense of justice.* This arises from their deficiency in the power of reasoning already referred to, and reflection, but is also partly due to the fact that Nature has not destined them, as the weaker sex, to be dependent on strength but on cunning; this is why they are instinctively crafty, and have an ineradicable tendency to lie. For as lions are furnished with claws and teeth, elephants with tusks, boars with fangs, bulls with horns, and the cuttlefish with its dark, inky fluid, so Nature has provided woman for her protection and defence with the faculty of dissimulation, and all the power which Nature has given to man in the form of bodily strength and reason has been conferred on woman in this form. Hence, dissimulation is innate in woman and almost as characteristic of the very stupid as of the clever. Accordingly, it is as natural for women to dissemble at every opportunity as it is for those animals to turn to their weapons when they are attacked; and they feel in doing so that in a certain measure they are only making use of their rights. Therefore a woman who is perfectly truthful and does not dissemble is perhaps an impossibility. This is why they see through dissimulation in others so easily; therefore it is not advisable to attempt it with them. From the fundamental defect that has been stated, and all that it involves, spring falseness, faithlessness, treachery, ungratefulness, and so on. In a court of justice women are more often found guilty of perjury than men. It is indeed to be generally questioned whether they should be allowed to take an oath at all. From time to time there are repeated cases everywhere of ladies, who want for nothing, secretly pocketing and taking away things from shop counters.

Nature has made it the calling of the young, strong, and handsome men to look after the propagation of the human race; so that the species may not degenerate. This is the firm will of Nature, and it finds its expression in the passions of women. This law surpasses all others in both age and power. Woe then to the man who sets up rights and interests in such a way as to make them stand in the way of it; for whatever he may do or say, they will, at the first sig-nificant onset, be unmercifully annihilated. For the secret, unformulated, nay, unconscious but innate moral of woman is: *We are justified in deceiving those who, because they care a little for us,—that is to say for the individual,—imagine they have obtained rights over the species. The constitution, and consequently the welfare of the species, have been put into our hands and entrusted to our care through the medium of the next generation which proceeds from us; let us fulfil our duties conscientiously.*

But women are by no means conscious of this leading principle *in abstracto*, they are only conscious of it *in concreto*, and have no other way of expressing it than in the manner in which they act when the opportunity arrives. So that their conscience does not trouble them so much as we imagine, for in the darkest depths of their hearts they are conscious that in violating their duty towards the individual they have all the better fulfilled it towards the species, whose claim upon them is infinitely greater. (A fuller explanation of this matter may be found in vol. ii., ch. 44, in my chief work, *The World as Will and Representation*.)

Because women in truth exist entirely for the propagation of the race, and their destiny ends here, they live more for the species than for the individual, and in their hearts take the affairs of the species more seriously than those of the individual. This gives to their whole being and character a certain frivolousness, and altogether a certain tendency which is fundamentally different from that of man; and this it is which develops that discord in married life which is so prevalent and almost the normal state.

It is natural for a feeling of mere indifference to exist between men, but between women it is actual enmity. This is due perhaps to the fact that *odium figulinum* [lit. "the jealousy of a tradesman"] in the case of men, is limited to their everyday affairs, but with women embraces the whole sex; since they have only one kind of business. Even when they meet in the street, they look at each other like Guelphs and Ghibellines. And it is quite evident when two women first make each other's acquaintance that they exhibit more constraint and dissimulation than two men placed in similar circumstances. This is why an exchange of compliments between two women is much more ridiculous than between two men. Further, while a man will, as a rule, address others, even those inferior to himself, with a certain feeling of consideration and humanity, it is unbearable to see how proudly and disdainfully a lady of rank will, for the most part, behave towards one who is in a lower rank (not employed in her service) when she speaks to her. This may be because differences of rank are much more precarious with women than with us, and consequently more quickly change their line of conduct and elevate them, or because while a hundred things must be weighed in our case, there is only one to be weighed in theirs, namely, with which man they have found favour; and again, because of the one-sided nature of their vocation they stand in closer relationship to each other than men do; and so it is they try to render prominent the differences of rank.

It is only the man whose intellect is clouded by his sexual instinct that could give that stunted, narrow-shouldered, broad-hipped, and short-legged race the name of *the fair sex*; for the entire beauty of the sex is based on this instinct. One would be more justified in calling them the *unaesthetic* sex than the beautiful. Neither for music, nor for poetry, nor for fine art have they any real or true sense and susceptibility; and it is mere mockery on their part, in their desire to please, if they affect any such thing.

This makes them incapable of taking a purely objective interest in anything, and the reason for it is, I fancy, as follows. A man strives to get *direct* mastery over things either by understanding them or by compulsion. But a woman is always and everywhere driven to *indirect* mastery, namely through a man; all her *direct* mastery being limited to him alone. Therefore it lies in woman's nature to look upon everything only as a means for winning man, and her interest in anything else is always a simulated one, a mere roundabout way to gain her ends, consisting of coquetry and pretence. Hence Rousseau said, *Les femmes, en général, n'aiment aucun art, ne se connoissent à aucun et n'ont aucun génie* ["Women in general do not like any art, do not know themselves and have no genius"]. Every one who can see through a sham must have found this to be the case. One need only watch the way they behave at a concert, the opera, or the play; the childish simplicity, for instance, with which they keep on chattering during the finest passages in the greatest masterpieces. If it is true that the Greeks forbade women to go to the play, they acted in a right way; for they would at any rate be able to hear something. In our day it would be more appropriate to substitute *taceat mulier in theatro* ["Let the woman be quiet in the theatre"] for *taceat mulier in ecclesia* ["Let the woman be quiet in church"];

and this might perhaps be put up in big letters on the curtain.

Nothing different can be expected of women if it is borne in mind that the most eminent of the whole sex have never accomplished anything in the fine arts that is really great, genuine, and original, or given to the world any kind of work of permanent value. This is most striking in regard to painting, the technique of which is as much within their reach as within ours; this is why they pursue it so industriously. Still, they have not a single great painting to show, for the simple reason that they lack that objectivity of mind which is precisely what is so directly necessary in painting. They always stick to what is subjective. For this reason, ordinary women have no susceptibility for painting at all: for *natura non facet saltum* ["Nature does not make a leap"]. And Huarte, in his book which has been famous for three hundred years, *Examen de ingenios para las scienzias*, contends that women do not possess the higher capacities. Individual and partial exceptions do not alter the matter; women are and remain, taken altogether, the most thorough and incurable philistines; and because of the extremely absurd arrangement which allows them to share the position and title of their husbands they are a constant stimulus to his ignoble ambitions. And further, it is because they are philistines that modern society, to which they give the tone and where they have sway, has become corrupted. As regards their position, one should be guided by Napoleon's maxim, *Les femmes n'ont pas de rang* ["Women have no rank"]; and regarding them in other things, Chamfort says very truly: *Elles sont faites pour commercer avec nos faiblesses avec notre folie, mais non avec notre raison. Il existe entre elles et les hommes des sympathies d'épiderme et très-peu de sympathies d'esprit d'âme et de caractère* ["They are made to trade with out weaknesses, with iur madness, but not with our reason. There exists between them and men a shared feeling that is skin-deep and very little sympathy of spirit, soul and character"]. They are the *sexus sequior*, the second sex in every respect, therefore their weaknesses should be spared, but to treat women with extreme reverence is ridiculous, and lowers us in their own eyes. When nature divided the human race into two parts, she did not cut it exactly through the middle! The difference between the positive and negative poles, according to polarity, is not merely qualitative but also quantitative. And it was in this light that the ancients and people of the East regarded woman; they recognised her true position better than we, with our old French ideas of gallantry and absurd veneration, that highest product of Christian-Teutonic stupidity. These ideas have only served to make them arrogant and imperious, to such an extent as to remind one at times of the holy apes in Benares, who, in the consciousness of their holiness and inviolability, think they can do anything and everything they please.

In the West, the woman, that is to say the "lady," finds herself in a *fausse position*; for woman, rightly named by the ancients *sexus sequior*, is by no means fit to be the object of our honour and veneration, or to hold her head higher than man and to have the same rights as he. The consequences of this *fausse position* are sufficiently clear. Accordingly, it would be a very desirable thing if this Number Two of the human race in Europe were assigned her nat-

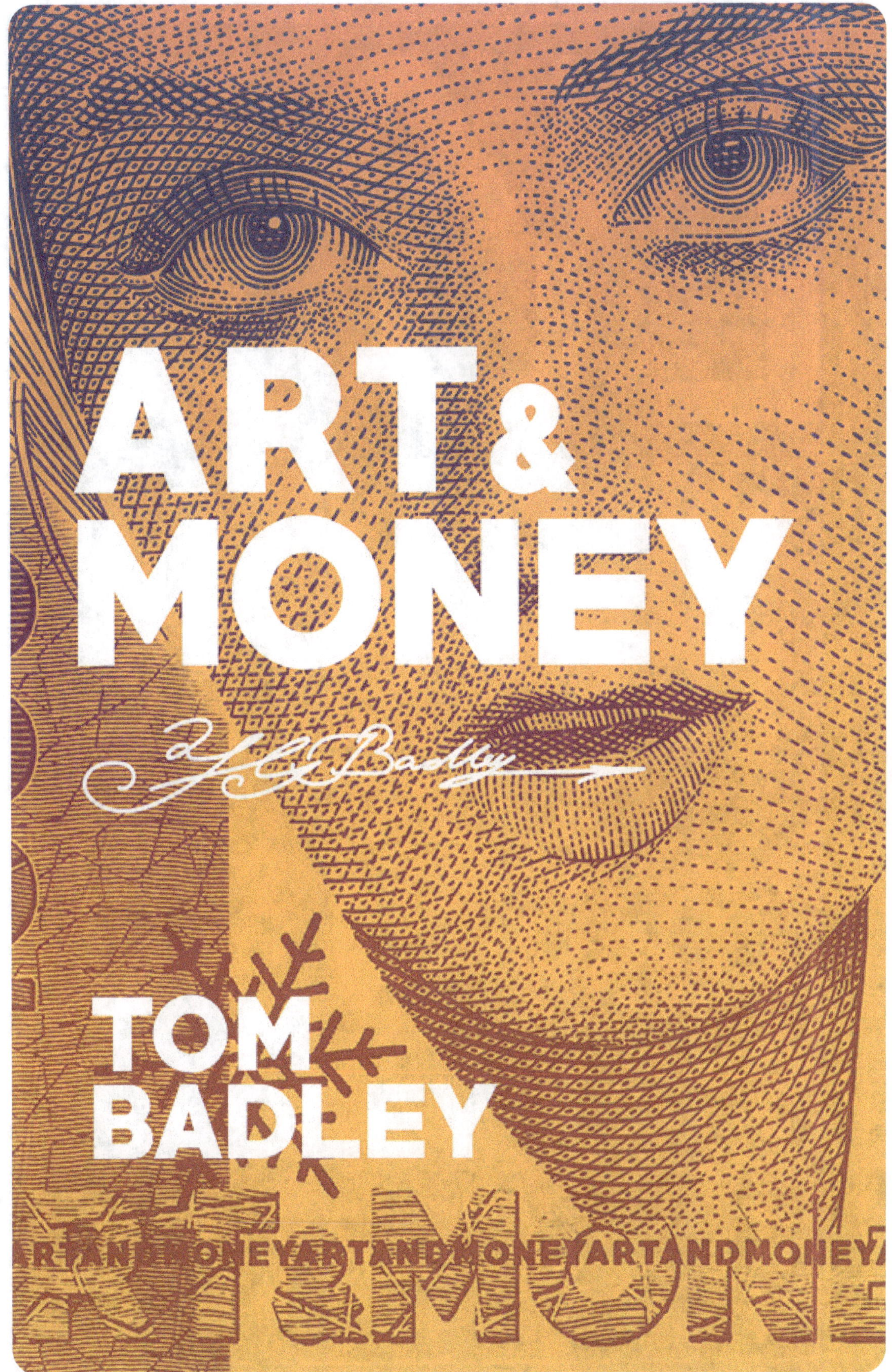

ART &
MONEY
TOM
BADLEY

FIAT LUX

~ a novel by ~
William du Jour

ural position, and the lady-grievance got rid of, which is not only ridiculed by the whole of Asia, but would have been equally ridiculed by Greece and Rome. The result of this would be that the condition of our social, civil, and political affairs would be incalculably improved. The Salic law would be unnecessary; it would be a superfluous truism. The European lady, strictly speaking, is a creature who should not exist at all; but there ought to be housekeepers, and young girls who hope to become such; and they should be brought up not to be arrogant, but to be domesticated and submissive. It is exactly because there are ladies in Europe that women of a lower standing, that is to say, the greater majority of the sex, are much more unhappy than they are in the East. Even Lord Byron says, *Thought of the state of women under the ancient Greeks—convenient enough. Present state, a remnant of the barbarism of the chivalric and feudal ages—artificial and unnatural. They ought to mind home—and be well fed and clothed—but not mixed in society. Well educated, too, in religion—but to read neither poetry nor politics—nothing but books of piety and cookery. Music— drawing—dancing—also a little gardening and ploughing now and then. I have seen them mending the roads in Epirus with good success. Why not, as well as hay-making and milking?*

In our part of the world, where monogamy is in force, to marry means to halve one's rights and to double one's duties. When the laws granted woman the same rights as man, they should also have given her a masculine power of reason. On the contrary, just as the privileges and honours which the laws decree to women surpass what Nature has meted out to them, so is there a proportional decrease in the number of women who really share these privileges; therefore the remainder are deprived of their natural rights in so far as the others have been given more than Nature accords.

For the unnatural position of privilege which the institution of monogamy, and the laws of marriage which accompany it, assign to the woman, whereby she is regarded throughout as a full equivalent of the man, which she is not by any means, cause intelligent and prudent men to reflect a great deal before they make so great a sacrifice and consent to so unfair an arrangement. Therefore, whilst among polygamous nations every woman finds maintenance, where monogamy exists the number of married women is limited, and a countless number of women who are without support remain over; those in the upper classes vegetate as useless old maids, those in the lower are reduced to very hard work of a distasteful nature, or become prostitutes, and lead a life which is as joyless as it is void of honour. But under such circumstances they become a necessity to the masculine sex; so that their position is openly recognised as a special means for protecting from seduction those other women favoured by fate either to have found husbands, or who hope to find them. In London alone there are 80,000 prostitutes. Then what are these women who have come too quickly to this most terrible end but human sacrifices on the altar of monogamy? The women here referred to and who are placed in this wretched position are the inevitable counterbalance to the European lady, with her pretensions and arrogance. Hence polygamy is a real benefit to the female sex, taking it *as a whole*. And, on the other hand, there is no reason why a man whose wife suffers from chronic illness, or remains barren, or has gradually become too old for him, should not take a second. Many people become converts to Mormonism for the precise reasons that they condemn the unnatural institution of monogamy. The conferring of unnatural rights upon women has imposed unnatural duties upon them, the violation of which, however, makes them unhappy. For example, many a man thinks marriage unadvisable as far as his social standing and monetary position are concerned, unless he contracts a brilliant match. He will then wish to win a woman of his own choice under different conditions, namely, under those which will render safe her future and that of her children. Be the conditions ever so just, reasonable, and adequate, and she consents by giving up those undue privileges which marriage, as the basis of civil society, alone can bestow, she must to a certain extent lose her honour and lead a life of loneliness; since human nature makes us dependent on the opinion of others in a way that is completely out of proportion to its value. While, if the woman does not consent, she runs the risk of being compelled to marry a man she dislikes, or of shrivelling up into an old maid; for the time allotted to her to find a home is very short. In view of this side of the institution of monogamy, Thomasius's profoundly learned treatise, *de Concubinatu*, is well worth reading, for it shows that, among all nations, and in all ages, down to the Lutheran Reformation, concubinage was allowed, nay, that it was an institution, in a certain measure even recognised by law and associated with no dishonour.

And it held this position until the Lutheran Reformation, when it was recognised as another means for justifying the marriage of the clergy; whereupon the Catholic party did not dare to remain behindhand in the matter.

It is useless to argue about polygamy, it must be taken as a fact existing everywhere, the *mere regulation* of which is the problem to be solved. Where are there, then, any real monogamists? We all live, at any rate for a time, and the majority of us always, in polygamy. Consequently, as each man needs many women, nothing is more just than to let him, nay, make it incumbent upon him to provide for many women. By this means woman will be brought back to her proper and natural place as a subordinate being, and *the lady*, that monster of European civilisation and Christian-Teutonic stupidity, with her ridiculous claim to respect and veneration, will no longer exist; there will still be *women*, but no *unhappy women*, of whom Europe is at present full. The Mormons' standpoint is right.

In India no woman is ever independent, but each one stands under the control of her father or her husband, or brother or son, in accordance with the law of Manu.

It is certainly a revolting idea that widows should sacrifice themselves on their husband's dead body; but it is also revolting that the money which the husband has earned by working diligently for all his life, in the hope that he was working for his children, should be wasted on her paramours. *Medium tenuere beati* ["Blessed they who take the middle course"]. The first love of a mother, as that of animals and men, is purely *instinctive*, and consequently ceases when the child is no longer physically helpless. After that, the first love should be reinstated by a love based on habit and reason; but this often does not appear, especially where the mother has not loved the father. The love of a father for his children is of a different nature and more sincere; it is founded on a recognition of his own inner self in the child, and is therefore metaphysical in its origin.

In almost every nation, both of the new and old world, and even among the Hottentots, property is inherited by the male descendants alone; it is only in Europe that one has departed from this. That the property which men have with difficulty acquired by long-continued struggling and hard work should afterwards come into the hands of women, who, in their want of reason, either squander it within a short time or otherwise waste it, is an injustice as great as it is common, and it should be prevented by limiting the right of women to inherit. It seems to me that it would be a better arrangement if women, be they widows or daughters, only inherited the money for life secured by mortgage, but not the property itself or the capital, unless there lacked male descendants. It is men who make the money, and not women; therefore women are neither justified in having unconditional possession of it nor capable of administrating it. Women should never have the free disposition of wealth, strictly so-called, which they may inherit, such as capital, houses, and estates. They need a guardian always; therefore they should not have the guardianship of their children under any circumstances whatever. The vanity of women, even if it should not be greater than that of men, has this evil in it, that it is directed on material things—that is to say, on their personal beauty and then on tinsel, pomp, and show. This is why they are in their right element in society. This it is which makes them inclined to be *extravagant*, especially since they possess little reasoning power. Accordingly, an ancient writer says, Γυνη το συνολον ἐστι δαπανηρον φυσει ["Women are expensive"]. Men's vanity, on the other hand, is often directed on non-material advantages, such as intellect, learning, courage, and the like. Aristotle explains in the *Politics* the great disadvantages which the Spartans brought upon themselves by granting too much to their women, by allowing them the right of inheritance and dowry, and a great amount of freedom; and how this contributed greatly to the fall of Sparta. May it not be that the influence of women in France, which has been increasing since Louis XIII.'s time, was to blame for that gradual corruption of the court and government which led to the first Revolution, of which all subsequent disturbances have been the result? In any case, the false position of the female sex, so conspicuously exposed by the existence of the "lady," is a fundamental defect in our social condition, and this defect, proceeding from the very heart of it, must extend its harmful influence in every direction. That woman is by nature intended to obey is shown by the fact that every woman who is placed in the unnatural position of absolute independence at once attaches herself to some kind of man, by whom she is controlled and governed; this is because she requires a master. If she, is young, the man is a lover; if she is old, a priest.

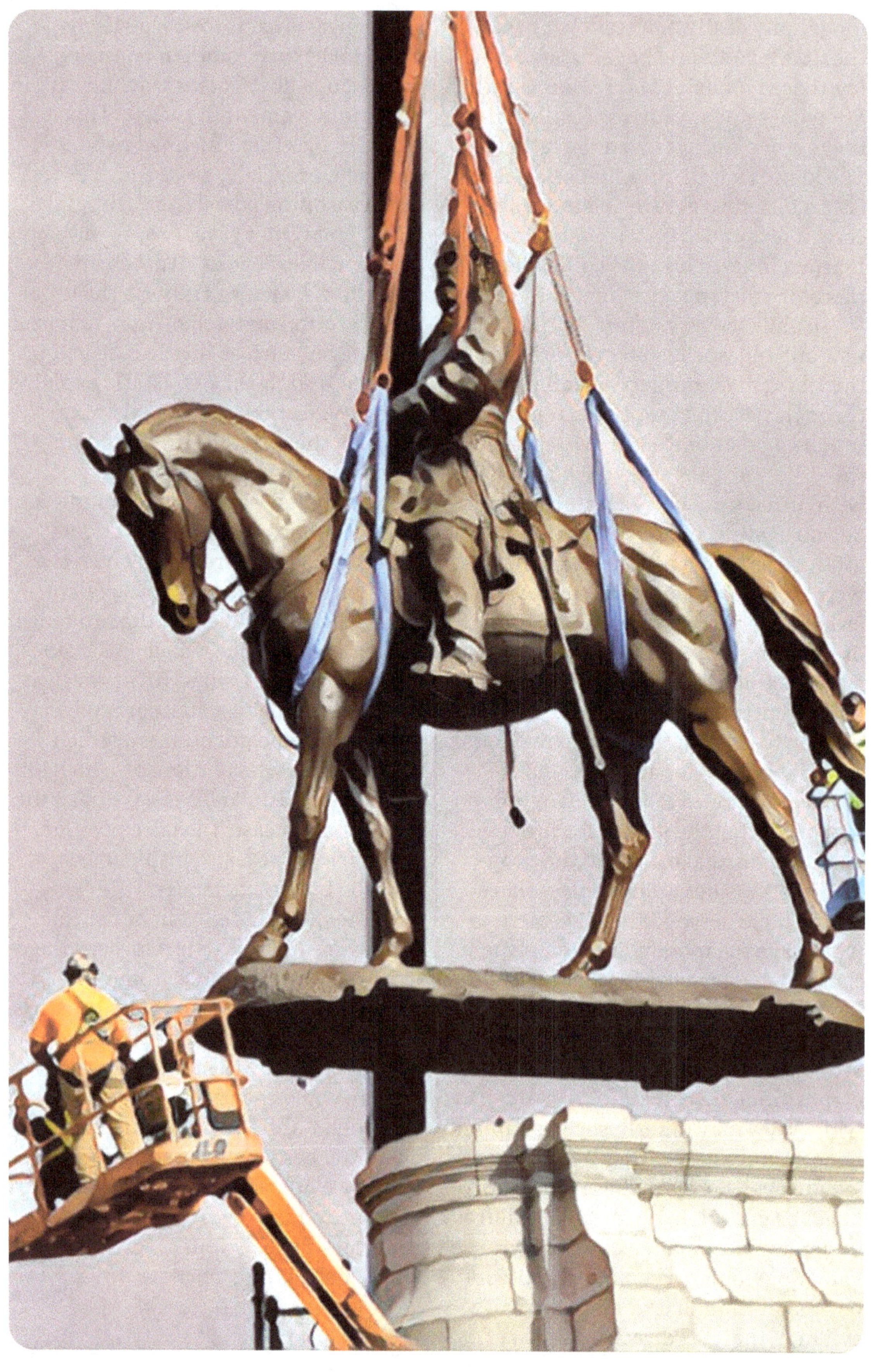

THE BATTLE FOR AMERICA'S SACRED SYMBOLS

essay by HAMILTON WESLEY ELLIS

The symbols of America's illustrious past hold great power for its present and future, which is why the nation's enemies must destroy them, at all cost...

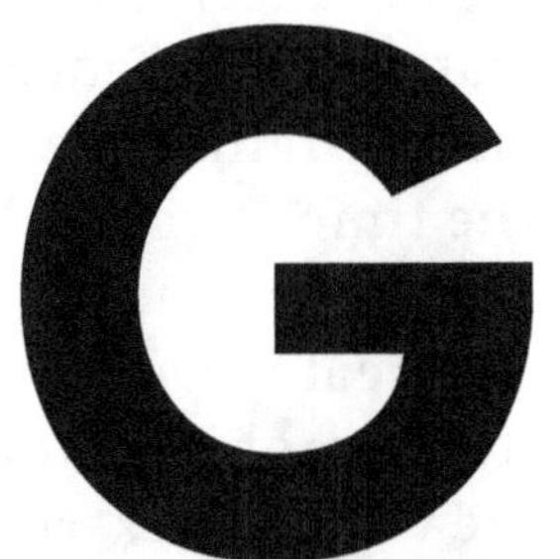

Gene Wolfe once wrote, "We believe that we invent symbols. The truth is, they invent us. We are their creatures, shaped by their hard defining edges." If Wolfe is correct, then we are doubly-defined by symbols that commemorate history. We use them to acclimate ourselves to our current environs, and as a temporal link to the figures and events that brought us here.

The ghouls of posthuman globalism are all too aware of the power of symbols. That's why they work to topple any monument that cannot conform to their graven narrative and erect in their stead repulsive new altars to the stultified gods of moral pedantry. Given their way, these self-appointed moral arbiters will festoon the land with their debased spectacles until our collective consciousness becomes so deprived of oxygen we dissociate from the last vestiges of our cultural past.

To this end, they're razing the names and likenesses of the men who fought for the Confederate States of America during the American Civil War. In their place, we're treated to their new idols; law-giving tentacled abortion demons, MLK memorials that vaguely resemble scatalogical pornography, and of course, innumerable depictions of the Apotheosis of George Floyd. Paul Fahrenheidt is one of a growing number of people who are tired of this sculptural terrorism.

Our perception of the past is integral to our conception of

who we are. Do we have the intellectual maturity and fortitude to accept history as a rich tapestry that contains good, bad, and ugly in each thread, or do we require past events be relayed to us in the form of a simple grade school-tier morality play? If we are unable to even attempt to understand the complexities of the past, we lack the ability to master our own future. The struggle here is far deeper than a quarrel to re-litigate battles that were decided over a century and half ago. It's a symbolic war for reality. Every time a historic monument is toppled, we are incrementally removed further from the truth. Every new altar that is erected in its stead comprises a looming threat to enshroud us all in a veil of lies.

I got a firsthand glimpse of the realities of monumental revision when they dug up General Nathan Bedford Forrest. I was in Memphis helping a friend clean out his downtown garage and as I was walking to a gas station to buy some drinks, I heard a racket coming from a nearby park. Turns out the din was a group of proud white southerners brandishing signs on one side of a chain link fence while a proud black lady was addressing a crowd of news reporters on the other side. Ebony and Ivory in perfect disharmony, broadcast for consumption on the evening news: a quintessentially Memphis happening.

Despite all the hubbub I witnessed, Forrest's removal from the city limits was a *fait accompli*. His statues had been removed from the city years ago, and the park that once bore his name had also been renamed. The only thing left for the city to do was disgorge the remains of the man himself. The late general and his wife, Mary Anne Montgomery, had rested safely in the same place for 144 years thanks to a law that required the State Historical Commission to grant permission for any disturbance to graves on state-owned land. The Historical Commission was stalwart in preserving the graves, but the Shelby County Commission finally figured an end run around the rule. One of the county commissioners created a nonprofit to purchase the land containing the graves, ensuring the Wizard of the Saddle and his wife would be disinterred, then reburied at the National Confederate Museum in Colombia, Tennessee.

At the time, I was ambivalent about Forrest's removal. He was a figure of great import inextricably linked to Memphis history, but I could see why a black-run city would take umbrage at being the final resting place of such an indomitable personage. Truth be told, if Nathan Bedford Forrest were to survey modern-day Memphis, he would likely elect to be buried elsewhere as well. The fact the city removed him came as a surprise to no one. History in Tennessee is much like the interminable rivers that lace the state. They twist, they turn, they ultimately reach a foreseeable conclusion based on surrounding topography. History is quite a different thing in the Old Dominion. If history in Tennessee is a river, in Virginia it's a city of marble. She is the most regal Southern state. Her soil reared our boldest, most brilliant founders. That soil was soaked in founding blood to birth our nation. Paul Fahrenheidt is a Virgin-

"THEIR DREAM IS TO MAKE ABERRANCY THE NORM, AND THEY ARE TRYING TO ACHIEVE THIS THROUGH MISEDUCATION"

ian.

He's also an author. Earlier this year, he published *A Country Squire's Notebook*, a collection of short stories that evince his unique American Mythos. Fahrenheidt observes the fractious nature of modern existence through a sophisticated lens in his writing. He weaves observations of the present with deep historical threads: a stark departure from the single-serving hot take milieu that confronts us so often today. He writes with forethought and sincerity, and is fearless with analysis of societal decay from the periphery of his Orange County estate. He explains eloquently that he describes himself as a liberal because he believes liberalism is the most suitable paradigm for a people as dynamic as the Sons of Aryas. His work runs the gamut from personal observation to tales of the postbellum era of American industrial giants. Recently though, this man of letters has been compelled to action. The locus of Mr. Fahrenheidt's concern: a dead horse's headstone.

The horse in question was a gelding named Traveller. That's two "l's" in the British style, a moniker befitting a steed of Virginia. On June 14, 2023, Washington and Lee University removed the headstone from the grave of the gray American Saddlebred, making the horse the latest victim of the destructive trend to oblite-rate, deface, and replace every single monument that fails to conform to a superficial and ignorant historical narrative. What, you ask, is the horse's crime? While there is no way to conclusively discern Traveller's thoughts on Emancipation or the root causes of the Civil War, we do know that he was General Robert E. Lee's favorite horse, and for that guilty association, he had to pay. Washington and Lee removed Traveller's original headstone, because it dared mention he was Lee's favorite horse. The irony of a university bearing Lee's name removing mention of it on a campus monument is lost on no one but the current campus administration.

"Washington and Lee is very near and dear to my heart, being a Virginian who deeply admires and seeks to emulate Lee. The attack on Traveller, a literal HORSE, seemed so insanely petty it was a good attack vector," says Fahrenheidt. He coordinated a robust response to the school's act of erasure. His clarion call was simple and powerful, "If those above us fail to preserve our history, then we must." He went as far to propose combatting the destruction of historical monuments with 3-D printers and Quickrete, answering the removal of old statues with a guerilla campaign to dot the land with high-tech reproductions. This might not be the hill Fahrenheidt dies on, but he has been admirably resolute in his efforts to swing the pendulum back towards status quo ante. Fahrenheidt's activism is also a test of the strength of liberal institutions. Can they be induced to stop, or at least slow down and second-guess iconoclastic behavior if they face enough societal pressure?

Fahrenheidt's skirmish is part of a deeper conflict. Our monuments are high-value targets for those who would strip reality of its sinews and replace them with amoral purposelessness. French philosopher Jean Baudrilliard provided a sketch of the battlefield in his most famous work, *Simulacres et Simulation*, in which he diagnoses the postmodern trend of substituting truth with simulation via symbology. He contends that Modernism was an unbridled orgy of liberating force that pushed every social convention past the red line. As a result, every left-driven cultural occurrence in the orgy's wake has been a recurring simulation of the battles of Modernism, but with no real struggle or victory. Now we contend with Simulacrum, a world of disembodied symbols masquerading as substance, on an eternally-repeating loop. Acceleration is no longer possible in this world of simulation, for we accelerate in a void. Symbols have mutated from faithful representations of the real to distorted versions of it. They eventually become encoded meta-symbols before finally being completely untethered from reality. It's a deep, dark forest and not everyone is making it out in one piece.

Encounters with the Wraiths of the Simulacrum are unavoidable. They're the NPCs who have yet to encounter an official narrative they wouldn't stake their life on. They call their religion "Science" and they call religion "a dangerous threat to democracy." They let fly their ever-changing banner of Sodom alongside the Stars and Stripes. They launch beer ad campaigns featuring transsexual goblins and are completely aghast and befuddled when people decide they're suddenly no longer thirsty. They are worse than dishonest: they are true believers. They smell exactly what they're stepping in, and to them it has the aroma of roses. These are the denizens of Hyperreality, an all-encompassing simulation they cannot distinguish from the truth. They make art without beauty, promote sex without reproduction, and print money without value. Their dream is to make aberrancy the norm, and they are trying to achieve this through miseducation. They create a fictionalized version of the past to mold the future.

"To be honest, it's not even about the Civil War. The way I see it, it's a front of the wider Culture War against Christian White America. Union Commanders are used as totems to humiliate the Red State Americans, while Sherman and Grant are not understood," says Fahrenheidt. Deletionist propaganda larping as history serves us all poorly. The lives of great men are multifaceted, complex, and nuanced. The moral outrage at Lee for the unforgivable sin of once existing is an insult to anyone capable of thought. But for the Virginia Secession Convention of 1861, he would have commanded Federal forces at Lincoln's request. Lincoln himself was an avowed opponent of social and political equality between whites and blacks. Even Nathan Bedford Forrest lived a life that cannot be constrained by the bounds of a simplistic moral narrative. As a member of the Memphis City Council, he voted against Secession. These verities are intentionally discarded from the leftist moral fable, for they're off script. When a narrative goes from non-fiction to fiction, it trends from complexity to simplicity.

Simulacres et Simulation famously inspired the Matrix franchise. Baudrillard saw the films and hated them. "The Matrix is surely the kind of film about the matrix that the matrix would have been able to produce," he said. The Frenchman's boeuf was with the presentation. The fact the "real world" of Zion was visibly distinguishable from the machine-run facsimile of the matrix in the movie did not conform to his ideal of Simulacra. The simulation crumbles when juxtaposed with reality. Perfected Simulacrum is much like the Mandala effect: the absence of the Monopoly Man's monocle or the Fruit of The Loom cornucopia serves to mask the fact that these things no longer exist. The illusion looks tawdry when you use the truth as a reference. Take the real life behavior of the Matrix creators, the Wachowski brothers. After the success of the first movie, they eventually declared themselves the Wachowski sisters. This stunt gave us a more scathing contrast between reality and facade than their movies ever did. The real world could never confuse the Wachowski's with real women, because real women exist and we know what they look like. Simulation falls before truth like wheat before the scythe.

"The goal is to replace history with, essentially, an airport reality," says Fahrenheidt. He believes that this battle over monuments is a test of our fortitude and strength as a people. "It naturally follows from a culture which has become extremely risk averse to the point of persecution," he says. He's correct. A people who can be dispossessed of their past are both unable and unworthy to master their own future. If we cede this ground and condemn the memory of great men (and their horses) to ashes, we risk something far worse than the repetition of forgotten history. We condemn ourselves to confinement in a recursive loop of lies without meaning, without hope, and without end. For them, it's a war to control culture. For us, the battle is existential.

Paul Fahrenheidt has now become a symbol of the effort to preserve history from those who would destroy it. This is not to say he's taken a position in public debate, as such things no longer exist. What we endure now instead is projectile exchange between two parallel universes bound in enmity, heated by the friction of their irreconcilable differences. There is, nor can there be, discourse across the chasm. One side finds succor in the truths and ideals it holds dear while the other side tries to envelop it in *beau idéal* artifice. The war is symbolic, but the stakes are very real. Mr. Fahrenheidt is fighting the good fight. ◼

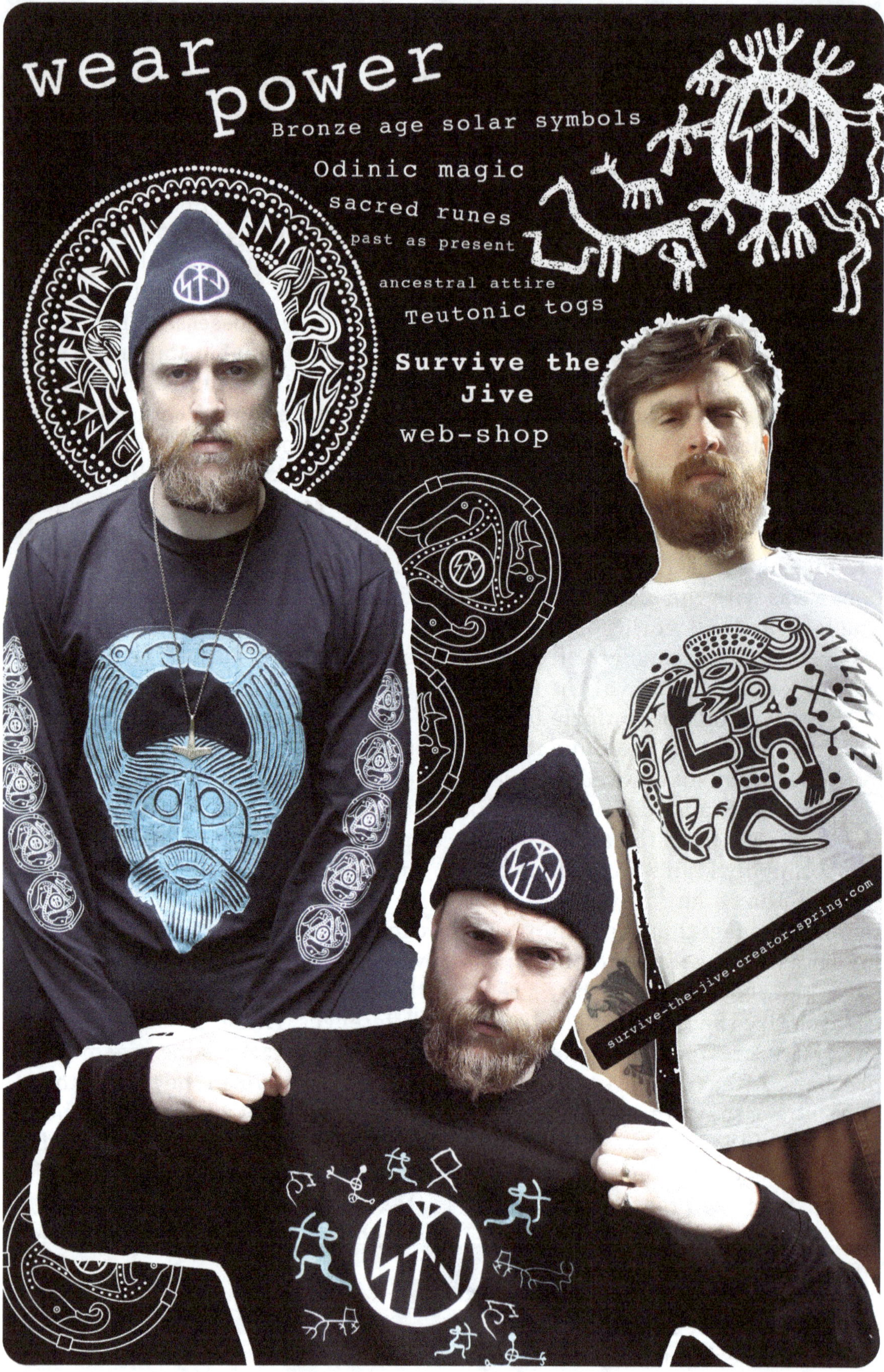

wear
power
Bronze age solar symbols
Odinic magic
sacred runes
past as present
ancestral attire
Teutonic togs
Survive the
Jive
web-shop
survive-the-jive.creator-spring.com

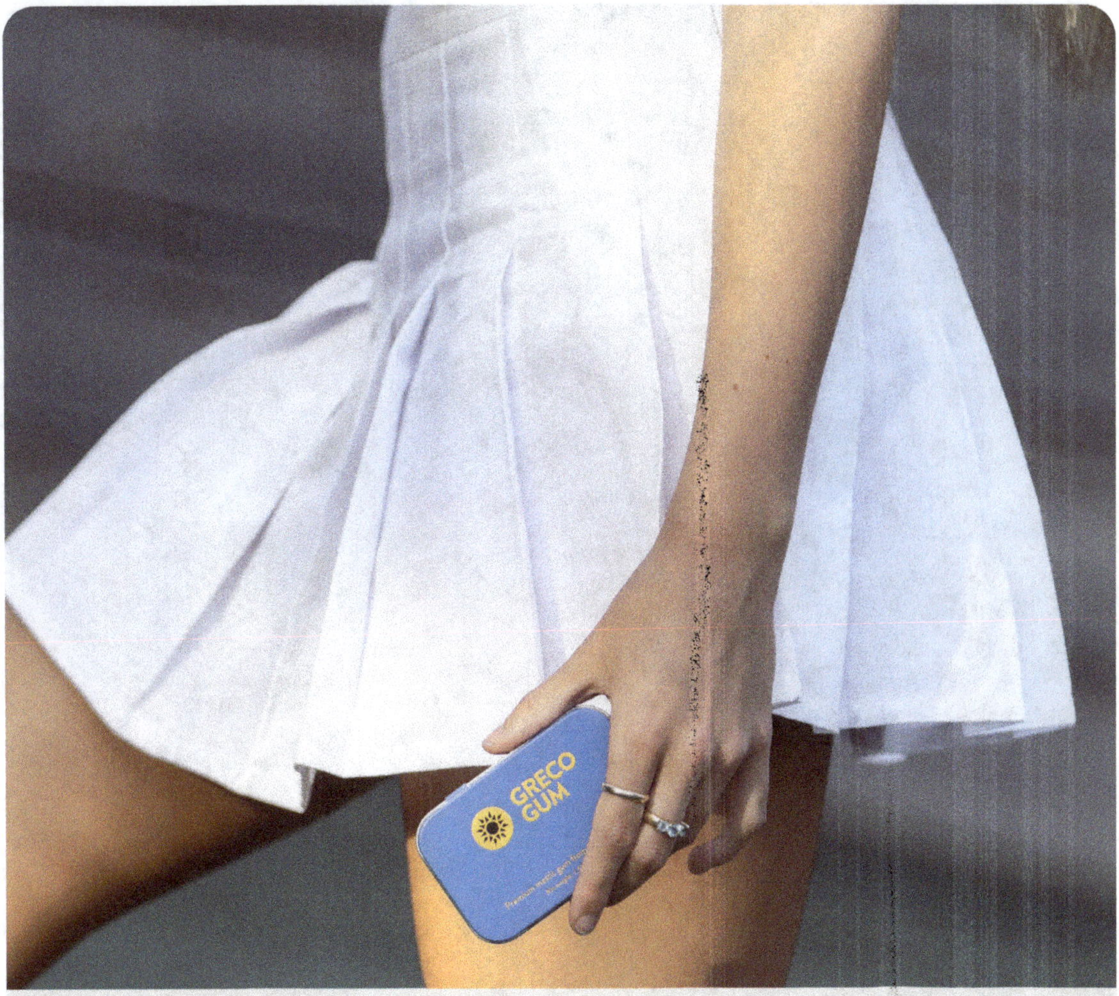

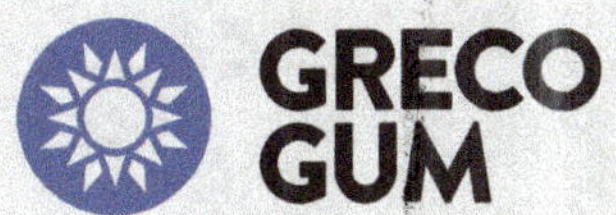

REMEMBER...
SHE WANTS TO
TOUCH IT.

(YOUR JAWLINE.)

GRECO
GUM

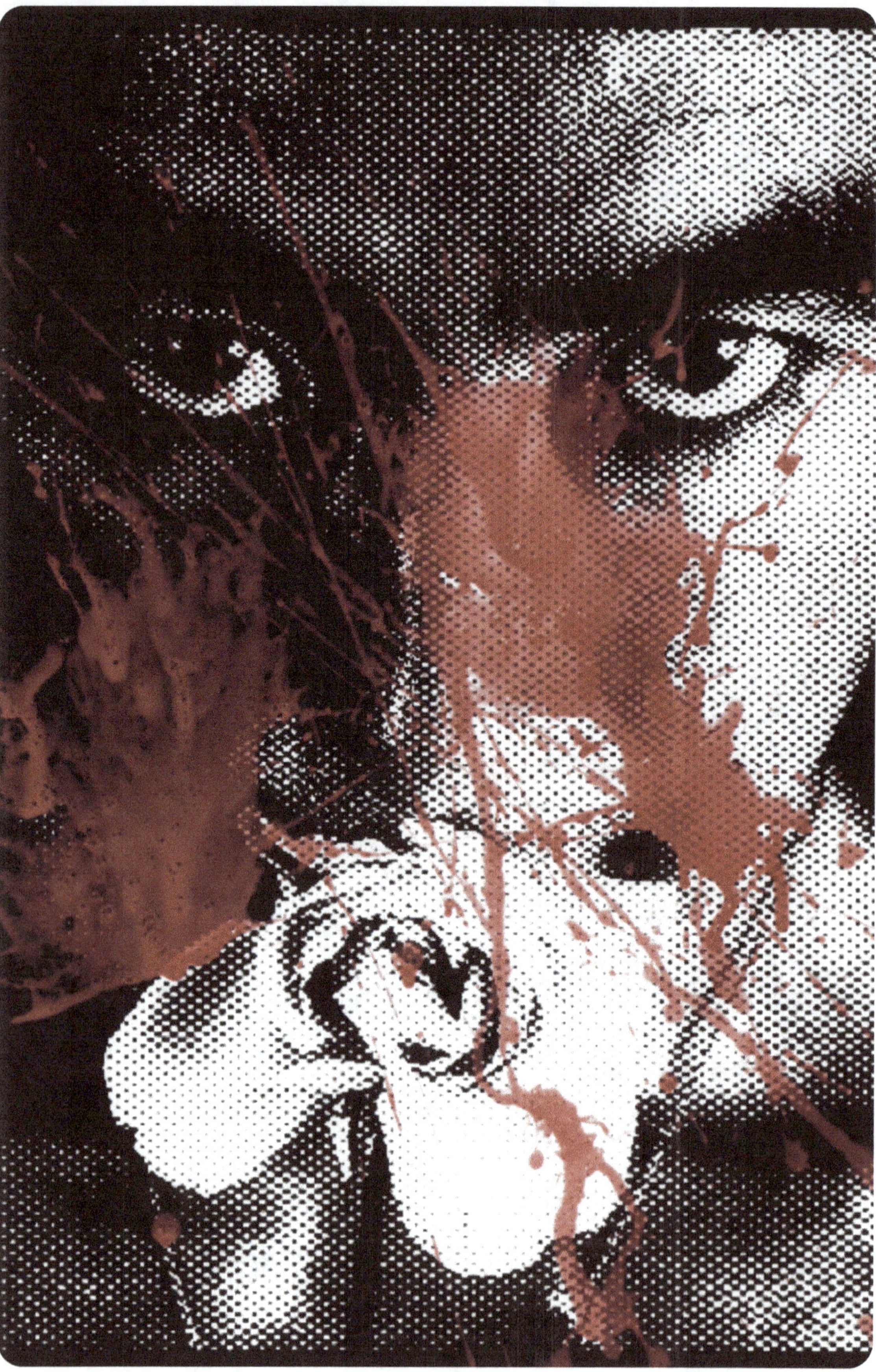

THE FIRST SEX

essay by CHOKODO SHUJIN

In Yukio Mishima's classic essay, we see the confrontation between traditional masculine heroism and the feminist desire to redefine and control it...

"**W**omen who have been married for two or three years usually come to the conclusion that men are stupid, simple, good-natured and, in short, children. Then, when women who have been married for more than ten years get together, they may not say it, but they will come to the conclusion that men are more or less scoundrels, liars, treacherous, and, in short, enigmatic. Finally, when wives who have reached their golden weddings gather together, the expression becomes much more moderate, back to the original conclusion, men are stupid, naïve, good-natured and, in short, children."

Thus begins Yukio Mishima's 1964 essay *Dai-ichi no Sei*, or "The First Sex", titled after Simone de Beauvoir's 1949 *The Second Sex*. In the form of a sprawling manifesto, Simone de Beauvoir asks, "What is woman?" Yukio Mishima, in response, asks, "What is man?" With his typical elegant yet rousing and inspired prose, he then delves into his exploration of the subject of masculinity in the modern era.

Mishima begins with his own observations of the behavior of modern women in relation to their various interactions with and general impressions of the opposite sex. "These conclusions are scientific enough," Mishima caustically says, "since most women are locked away in the sacred laboratory of their lifelong marriage, studying the poor male with great precision and care."

Upon examining these three conclusions drawn by modern urban women, it becomes apparent that the first and the third conclusion, although nearly identical in wording, are actually different in substance and content. The final conclusion is of course reached only after going through the second one, the vapid assertion that men are mentally and emotionally inferior to women. Fundamentally, he finds, modern women have little respect for men. In the end, the conclusion drawn by these patently Americanized housewives of Tokyo is simply that "men are bad." It is difficult to conceive of a more prescient statement, being that traditional masculinity has recently been categorized as a form of mental illness by the Diagnostic and Statistical Manual of Mental Disorders (DSM). Moreover, allegations of misogyny are sufficient grounds for dismissal from many places of employment, while misandry is casually accepted, or even encouraged and lauded. The simple and childish wording of the statement, too, "men are bad," reflects the simplistic and binary attitudes of those who supported such measures, who describe any outward demonstration of masculine characteristics as "toxic." Stoicism, heroism, individualism, restraint, and objectivity are mocked, while performative "caring," collectivism, and various patronizing forms of nurturing and faux-empathy as practiced by career women are all praised. To say that men are bad, of course, implies that women are good. These women do not want equality, but domination.

In the end, it is a woman's full-body expression of the very last possible admission: husbands should be treated like children, and women, who are natural nurturers, should be in charge. As Sonia Sotomayor said, cheered on by the mainstream media, "I would hope that a wise Latina woman with the richness of her experiences would more often than not reach a better conclusion than a white male who hasn't lived that life." I will let her quote speak for itself; no commentary is necessary. Such views, inappropriate as they may be, have become mainstream.

Beyond being merely ignorant of men's lives and motivations, women often seem to wilfully misunderstand men's actions and priorities. This behavior, too, has become unsettlingly mainstream – it is considered commendable even. American television and mass media perpetuate and then propagate such an image. Sitcoms and films typically feature the archetypes of a bumbling, incompetent husband, fat and guzzling beer, and his long-suffering wife, who saves him from whatever mishap he has gotten himself into. And yet I cannot fail to note that many modern female entertainers, in the guise of empowerment, celebrate their gluttony and sloth, and the obesity that follows. These women expect tall and handsome men to fall for them while damning and questioning the masculinity of any man who finds their repellent physiques and hysterical temperaments unattractive.

Even more extreme in its misandry is so-called prestige programming, in which men seem to solely exist to rape, abuse, and generally persecute women, or to offer their undiluted adulation to the brilliant and remarkably capable women who surround them. These are the two roles men are allowed to

"BEYOND BEING MERELY IGNORANT OF MEN'S LIVES AND MOTIVATIONS, WOMEN OFTEN SEEM TO WILFULLY MISUNDERSTAND MEN'S ACTIONS AND PRIORITIES"

play in the theaters of the American self-appointed elites. Strolling through various mainstream bookstores, I have seen that this abounds in novels as well. What is particularly disturbing is the number of these television programs and novels that are marketed towards young girls. The propagandization begins young.

Anecdotally, I have observed many women who take no interest in films or novels that feature male protagonists. "I just can't relate to them," a friend's wife said. It is an irony that would never occur to her that she insists upon her husband watching her preferred television shows with her, all of which have female protagonists, often teenage girls, and are heavily misandrist. Such women revel in their refusal to either understand or take the faintest interest in men, while expecting their husbands to find all aspects of the lives and the various problems of women to be endlessly fascinating. What is it about men, then, that women find so inscrutable?

"What is it that makes them go to war in the countryside to have a hard time when they have plenty of money, plenty of women, plenty of admiration from the world, and plenty of fun?" a hypothetical woman asks in Mishima's essay.

This is a lifelong process of recognition for women, but as Mishima says, from a male point of view, we can only say, "You don't get it, do you?"

Of course, here Mishima is implying something greater: that women largely and fundamentally do not understand the male instinct towards heroism.

When Lord Byron went abroad to support the Greek War of Independence, selling his estate to support a private army of thirty philhellene officers and about two hundred men, his faithful steward, who had served him for many years, said to him on the outbound ship, "I don't understand your lordship's feelings at all." Had Byron remained in England, he would have lived a life of privilege and luxury, a celebrated artist who wanted for nothing. Byron replied that he was honored to be misunderstood, for "[a] servant cannot understand the heart of a hero." This would have resonated with Mishima especially, a writer twice nominated for the Nobel Prize for Literature, who also founded a private army, the Tatenokai, or Shield Society, comprised mainly of young men from Waseda University. The Tatenokai was formed due to Mishima's alarm over the scale of leftist protests in Tokyo in 1968, although he vowed to stand against threats to Japan from both the left and the right.

"But nowadays, in a democracy, everyone is a servant," Mishima wrote in "The First Sex".

It seems that women are naturally democratic, which I have always maintained is a system very much like communism, at least in its present iteration. To simplify the matter perhaps too much, both systems involve governance by the masses. In a very democratic way, women typically believe that rather than be ruled by the elite, everyone should have a say, although as Orwell said in *Animal Farm*, some are more equal than others. Women typically shun the concept of nobility; anything but equality, or, lately, "equity," is unfashionable. And much like Lord Byron's devoted steward, women can rarely understand the psychology of a hero, instead looking at the daily lives of their husbands from a limited and myopic perspective. While Byron's steward was impressed though confused by this impulse to heroism, women tend to be repelled by it and aim to stifle or even extinguish this impulse.

"Every man is a hero," Mishima says. Indeed, the title of the first chapter of The First Sex is "All Men Are Heroes." He continues, "I say this as a man. It's just that the world's men are wrong. The only thing wrong with men in the world is that they try to make women see their heroism."

And modern women, upon seeing this heroism, are either threatened or repelled. For the modern feminist, the concept of heroism is viewed as inherently tied to patriarchal structures and ideals, which they describe as promoting a narrow and often exclusionary definition of strength and heroism. They argue that traditional heroes tend to reflect masculine qualities and reinforce traditional gender roles, sidelining or dismissing the experiences and contributions of women and marginalized groups, to use their jargon, which I cannot help but notice is strangely interchangeable with the jargon used by modern race baiters.

What then do these women advocate? The modern feminist might advocate a broader understanding of heroism that includes "diverse" perspectives and attributes. "Diverse," of course, is a euphemism for non-European and, increasingly, non-Asian. A "diverse" course in literature would not include Sōseki Natsume or Lu Xun, but instead whichever writers can be plucked from various developing countries, or American women and minorities. They celebrate what they describe as the courage and resilience of everyday people, shining a light on so-called individuals who challenge societal norms, fight for "social justice," and work towards destroying systems that they consider oppressive. It is a thoroughly Marxist doctrine.

In their eyes, heroism should encompass acts of compassion, empathy, and advocacy for communities that they define as marginalized. They emphasize collective action, community-building, and cooperation over individualistic notions of heroism. These feminists advocate narratives that explore "complex" characters – that is, characters who reflect their own experiences, preferences, and perspectives. Their diversity is remarkable in its homogeneity.

In "The First Sex", Mishima provides an anecdote in which a beautiful fashion model accidentally drove her car into a moat. Frightened and unable to swim, the young woman climbed onto the roof of her stranded car and shouted for help. Three men immediately appeared, jumped into the water, and rescued the woman. "...and we can only wonder how chivalry could have spread from Europe at the end of the

Middle Ages in the fifteenth century to Japan in the twentieth century," Mishima writes.

The three men in question were all men of great integrity. All three of them were unquestionably noble, not because they rescued the woman for some ulterior motive, not because any money or glory was at stake, but simply because they were "chivalrous heroes." This is one of many things that modern feminists are waging war against.

"Chivalry was a very cunning Western invention," writes Mishima. Indeed, it was chivalry that established an aesthetically pleasing image of the hero that was easy for women to understand. In the modern era, the hero has been reduced to an archetype. In fact, heroism is perhaps the most difficult idea for the modern woman to comprehend, but cunning chivalry is a successful adaptation of this ancient concept for the modern woman. As I described earlier, we see this cunning heroism on television in the form of the plucky female protagonist's adoring, obsequious, and non-threateningly handsome love interest.

"The men in the middle are real sissies," Mishima says quite candidly, describing these milquetoast figures. They know neither art nor action. "There is not a single heroic figure that women are concerned with, and heroes are all difficult figures for women to understand, from the ancient Japanese warrior Yamato Takeru-no-Mikoto, who achieved great deeds through the sacrifice of women, to the patriots of the late Tokugawa shogunate, who only knew women as merchant girls who fell to their knees."

In his long prose poem, "The Crowned Poet," Yojūrō Yasuda describes Takeru-no-Mikoto as such: "He was the epitome of one of Japan's finest warriors, and therefore also the epitome of a Japanese poet. Not only is it significant because he was a poet, but it is also significant because he was a warrior." Ryūnosuke Akutagawa, famous as a poet, writer, and aesthete, was also accomplished as a master of judo, and it was his contention that all artists should also be martial artists, and vice versa.

But for women, what matters is, essentially, emotion. To put it bluntly, the masculine principle is forever a mystery to women, just as the feminine principle is forever a mystery to men. And to understand the hero, the symbol of the masculine principle, a woman has no choice but to understand things in a woman's way. This leads to her interpreting the emotions and motivations of men as being essentially similar to her own, and drawing conclusions that are often vastly incorrect. As a result , she sees the man as some inferior and inscrutable "other," to use the modern parlance. When women weep, it is due to their profound empathy, yet when men weep, it is a failing, a weakness, in their eyes. In The Father, playwright August Strindberg addresses this, paraphrasing Shylock's famous monologue from *The Merchant of Venice*. "Yes, I am crying although I am a man. But has not a man eyes! Has not a man hands, limbs, senses, thoughts, passions? Is he not fed with the same food, hurt by the same weapons, warmed and cooled by the same summer and winter as a woman? If you prick us, do we not bleed? If you tickle us, do we not laugh? And if you poison us, do we not die? Why shouldn't a man complain, a soldier weep? Because it is unmanly?

THE MORALIST

Is It Ever Morally Acceptable For a Corded Ware Man To Visit an EEF Dolmen site?

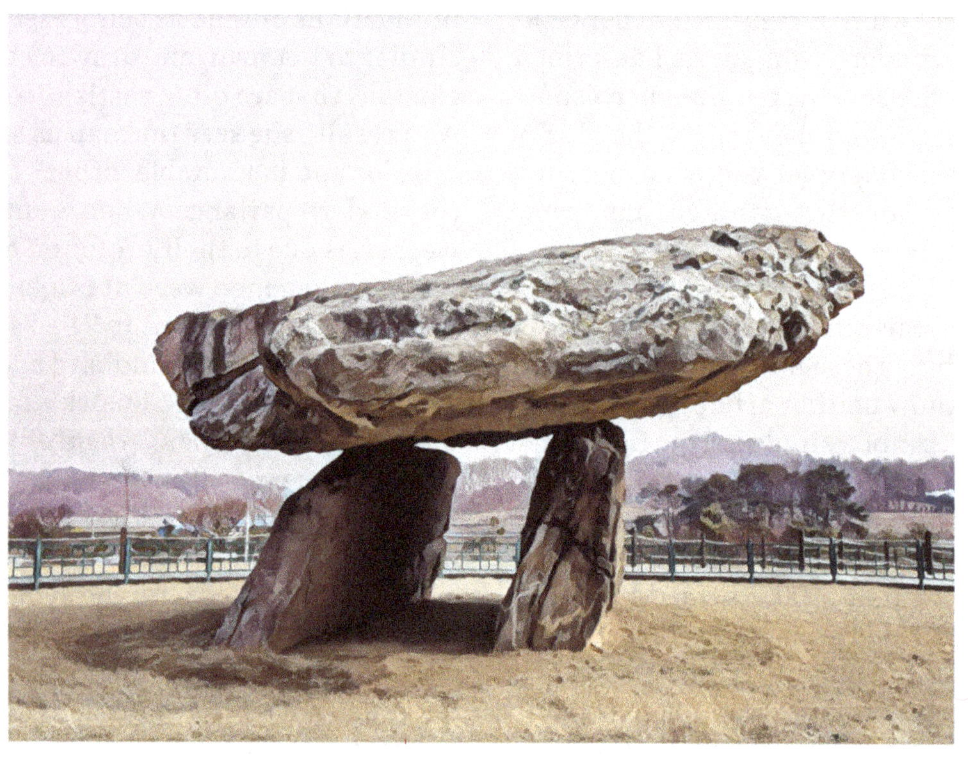

Why is it unmanly?"

Mishima describes the process of the typical feminine attempts to unravel a man's feelings as pulling the yarn from one place on a woollen doll when she finds a tear, finding a particular point of view when it comes undone, pulling the yarn out from that point of view, and then pulling the wool out again, and again, and again. They pull the yarn from the woollen doll until they eventually tear it to pieces, turning it into a mere ball of mangled yarn. "Poor men, they grow up in a storm from childhood. Subjected to ridicule, abuse, and criticism, they wear themselves out trying not to be the laughing stock of others. In the world of boys, the degree of respect depends on the development of secondary sexual characteristics."

In the world of boys, Mishima contends, the highest principle in the world is the test of heroism: to climb higher, to run faster, to prove one's physical and mental bravery. The most undeveloped aspect of such a competitive spirit remains even in adulthood, and although women are different in their love of physically strong men, and many women do not value strength to such a degree, most men without muscles envy men who are physically strong. This is no longer a question of merely being popular among women or not, but a remnant of the fierce competition for secondary sexual characteristics in the world of boys, and a lingering vestige of the near-extinct heroic type.

The pointlessness of the heroic struggle in the male world, even for muscular physique, still seems ridiculous to many modern women. The competition between women regarding appearance is vaguely similar to this, but modern women tend to decry any display of vanity, at least in public. This explains the popularity of designer sweatpants and nude lipstick, which are worn with the intention of impressing other women, rather than to appeal to men. This also explains the great number of overweight fashion models and pop singers. It is other women whose respect they seek, and in seeking this catty sort of respect, they often unflatteringly alter their appearances.

Let us return to the words of Mishima's anonymous Tokyo housewife.

"Men are stupid, simple, good-natured and, in short, children."

This is the conclusion of those who proclaim their superior empathy and emotional intelligence, the modern woman's substitute for physical vanity.

"But, wait a moment," Mishima says. The competition for women's appearances is solely a matter of the physical, but the heroics of men immediately pass through the physical realm and extend into the spiritual and metaphysical world. Although their basic motives are in essence childish, they reach the giants of the world of politics and economies, of philosophical thought and art, conquests, and war. In other words, a man's feet can lose ground more easily than a woman's. This is the privilege of men, as well as the source of all honor, Mishima writes. And this is something that should never be disparaged or discarded, regardless of the best attempts of modern progressives to destroy masculinity.

Originally published on Arktos.com as "Heroic Masculinity", where a second part can also be read.

VALIANT
NEWS
WE VALUE TRUTH
WWW.VALIANTNEWS.COM

WHERE OTHERS WON'T, WE
WILL
WILL
BASED MARKETING
@WILLtheagency
willtheagency.com

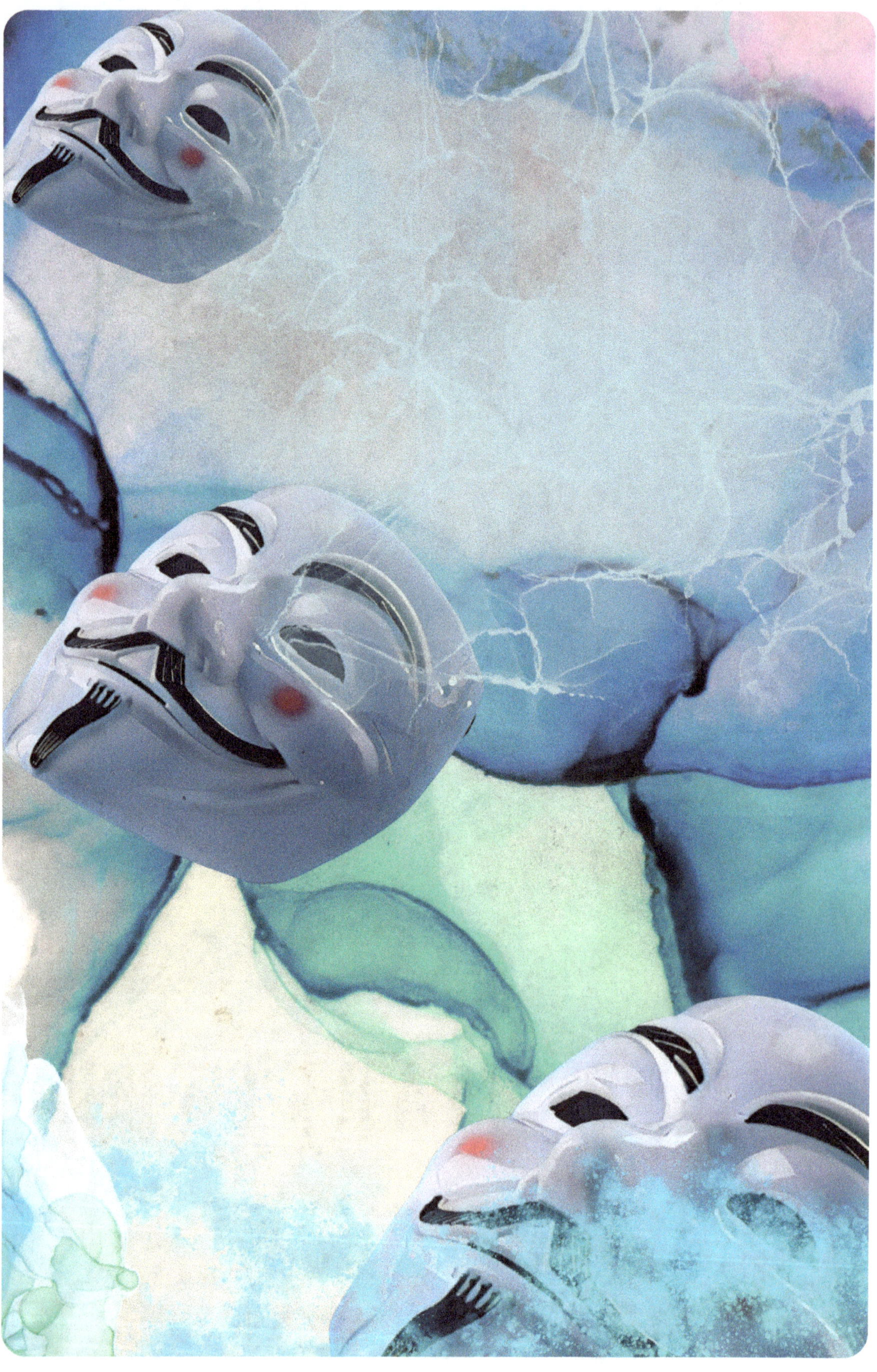

AN ACTUAL DEFENCE OF ANONYMITY

counterblast essay by RAW EGG NATIONALIST

Don't believe stinky interlopers who tell you internet anonymity only matters as a route to mainstream respectability. It's far more important than that...

I'm not entirely sure what a full philosophical or pragmatic defence of internet anonymity would look like, but one thing I do know is that neither would look anything like Mark Granza's "In defense of anons" (on the IM1776 website).

Granza's main concern in his piece seems to be to point out i) that there are different kinds of anonymity and ii) that the kind that really matters isn't anonymity at all; in fact, it's a form of pseudonymity, with ethical obligations attached to it that ensure the mask is worn in a responsible manner. Only a select few accounts qualify for this rare distinction, and the individuals behind them are the ones that have a shot at "landing a book deal" and taking their rightful place amid the ranks of the known. Fundamentally, it's these accounts that provide anonymous posting with whatever legitimacy it might have, and it's these accounts alone that can justify the excesses of those making use of anonymity for less productive reasons.

The mass of real anons, by contrast, are subject to less responsibility and behave with little to no restraint. We're talking about your cumgroypers, anime PFPs, classical statue heads, Mel Gibson Fans and so on. Their kind of anonymity is a necessary outlet for people who don't really have much of any value to say, and they certainly aren't likely to land a book deal (although I, for one, would love to know the backstory of Mel Gibson Fan 74). Given the current political climate, these people should have the right to say whatever it is they want to say without the risk of persecution – and the only way to ensure that is to allow them to speak out of impenetrable darkness, even if all they do is annoy other people. Nobody should have to risk their livelihood and personal relationships for the sake of posting that "shut up, bitch!" video of the Rock under a few tweets they don't like. These people can, of course, just be muted or blocked.

Before we get going, I think it's worth putting Jordan Peterson back in his box under the stairs. His beef with the anonymous community is personal, not philosophical. The increasingly shrill tone of his outbursts (demons! the dark tetrad!), and their increasingly strange prose-poetic form, is indicative of a man who is still unwell. Indeed, it's not even clear whether the "Jordan Peterson" we're interacting with on Twitter really is the man himself, or his daughter Mikhaila, who has taken on a role not unlike that of Jamie Spears in the months and years since her father's well-publicised battle with benzodiazepine addiction. Mikhaila has her own reasons to dislike anonymous posters on Twitter, not least of all the constant reminders of her three-day dalliance with a certain Emory Andrew Tate III in Romania.

And while we're at it, let's put Patrick Deneen in that box too. It's abundantly obvious why he wouldn't be happy with my friend Lomez for being published in *First Things*. The presence of anonymous Twitter posters in the hallowed pages of such a publication indicates a clear loss of control for tastemakers like Deneen, who believe that nobody, least of all a totally unknown quantity who hasn't been subject to their post-liberal gleichshaltung, should be allowed to slip through their networks of patronage. Heaven for-

bid, they might even have something important and compelling to say! A similar response was evident when I published my first essay with *American Mind*, a publication of the Claremont Institute, way back in early 2022. Not long after, Bill Kristol sent his attack poodles at the *Bulwark* after me. When Kristol tweeted the resulting hitpiece, which lamented the continuing moral "decay" at the Claremont Institute, his replies were full of people like "Ostrogothic King" force-feeding him the unpalatable truth: "Funny that someone named @babygravy9 has far more interesting things to say than anyone at the bulwark, the entire output of which seems to consist of indignant sputtering." Ouch.

So. When it comes to distinguishing between different kinds of anonymity, I can see what Mark Granza is trying to get at. There really is a difference between the typical behaviour of an anonymous account created solely for the purpose of trolling – and such things do exist – and the behaviour of an anonymous writer with a reputation, a large following and a bibliography of publications. I'm one of the latter; although I started out as the former, more or less (I had no social-media ambitions beyond having a bit of fun). There are many things that a troll account would readily do that I simply don't or won't do. Certain types of behaviour and certain topics of conversation are totally off-limits, and would have ended my Twitter career many months or even years ago if I'd decided to pursue them. In the beginning, I didn't do these things largely for reasons of temperament, but as my account and influence grew, this became a much more conscious thing for me. As things stand, I

"THE EXISTENTIAL NEED FOR SELF-CONCEALMENT IS AT THE BASE OF THE ENTIRE PHENOMENON OF ANONYMOUS TWITTER-POSTING"

have 170,000 followers and the ability to reach as far into the mainstream media as most named commentators.

Granza claims that the fundamental difference between "pseudonymous" and "anonymous" accounts is precisely the reputation accounts like mine have built up, which demands that the poster, whoever he or she may be, act with responsibility, or circumspection at the very least, rather than "screwing around". By contrast, a truly "anonymous" account has no ties to "any identifiable entity", giving it an ephemeral nature that permits a total lack of restraint if desired by the user. In support of this distinction, Granza cites a Youtube video involving a boring German man with a horrid ponytail and noodle arms that I just couldn't be bothered to watch. But I don't think we need a 50-minute lecture to understand that this distinction misses something fundamental that unites any and all accounts that operate under assumed identities.

Let's put to one side the linguistic quibble that to be anonymous by definition you would have to be "without name" (all anonymous accounts on Twitter are therefore pseudonymous accounts, technically, since they all have names). Consider the example of J.K. Rowling. When she decided to write again after finishing the Harry Potter series, she wanted to do so without the baggage of being "the Harry Potter woman". She wanted a clean slate. She chose, therefore, to write her Cormoran Strike series of crime novels under the gruffer *nom de plume* of Robert Galbraith. Initially, this was a well-kept secret, but pretty soon people found out. And what was the consequence? *Nothing.* Well, nothing bad, anyway. Rather, the discovery that Robert Galbraith was actually the Harry Potter woman provided massive exposure for a forgettable series of novels that would otherwise have been quickly forgotten, leading to more book sales, television dramatisations etc. Rowling might have wanted to maintain the fiction of being someone else, but she had absolutely no reason to fear being unmasked.

Pseudonymity in this case is just a distancing device, which may be adopted for a number of reasons but has nothing to do with ensuring the writer's sovereignty or personal safety. Other writers may choose pseudonyms because they simply don't have a writerly name. Bob Fudgepacker may be the best thriller writer in the continental United States, but with a name like that there's no chance he'll be taken seriously...

So not only is Granza's distinction between "pseudonymous" and "anonymous" accounts an affront to common sense, to our everyday understanding of what a pseudonymous writer is as opposed to someone trying to express themselves without any reference to who they really are, but it also minimises the fact that neither "pseudony-mous" nor "anonymous" posters want to be found out. Yes, a poster like me might have a reputation to preserve, but there's one thing that remains as off-the-table for me or Benjamin Braddock or Lafeyette Lee as it does for the lowliest shitposter and that's, of course, our actual names and faces. None of us wants, personally, to be an "identifiable entity", even if I may want people to know that, behind the mask, it's still the same handsome bodybuild-er who has published all those fasci-nating articles in *American Mind* and that wonderful new(-ish) book *The Eggs Benedict Option*. This existential need for self-concealment is at the base of the entire phenomenon of anonymous Twitter-posting, and no amount of definitional jerrymandering can change that.

And the thing is, as an anonymous writer builds a more prominent profile, the risks actually become greater, not smaller. The investment in anonymity grows, rather than shrinking. When I was "Turning Point Çatalhöyük" and had all of five followers, no journalist or Antifa scumbag had any interest in revealing my identity, in contrast to the situation today, where barely a day seems to pass without some fresh smear claiming I and others like me such as Bronze Age Pervert are mem-bers of the "Unabomber right" (kek!) or leaders of an emerging "raw food movement" that "may present the po-tential for violent consequences" (kek!). As silly as these claims may sound, the aim of the hitpieces they're drawn from is clearly to flag me and my more influ-ential friends as valid objects for inter-vention by the security services.

This hardly presents anonymous figures like me with an easy route to mainstream acceptance, even if we were looking for that, which most of us aren't. Thankfully, being anonymous now offers its own distinctive routes for influence and success largely on our own terms, not least of all self-publica-tion. *Bronze Age Mindset*, self-published through the Amazon KDP platform, has sold many tens of thousands of cop-ies since its release in 2018, regularly trouncing the most astroturfed estab-lishment authors in the classics, an-cient history and philosophy, including Mark Zuckerberg's fat sister Donna. As well as self-publishing books that have also sold many thousands of copies, I've created my own magazine, MAN'S WORLD, and website, which racked up more than 350,0000 hits during the release week of the latest issue.

It's impossible, I think, to write an honest account of internet anonymity today without mentioning the case of Douglass Mackey, a.k.a "Ricky Vaughn". His omission from Granza's "defense" is instructive. Ricky Vaughn, for those who don't know, was a prominent anonymous poster during the 2016 election cycle. Although it's difficult to quantify social media influence, Vaughn was widely identified as one of the key players in Trump's victory. The MIT Media Lab, for instance, named him ahead of NBC News, Stephen Col-bert, and the Drudge Report in its list of the top 150 influencers of the election. His memes and posts were regularly retweeted by some of the most impor-tant figures on the American right.

In 2018, the man behind the Ricky Vaughn account was revealed after Paul Nehlen, a congressional candidate, posted his name on Twitter. A gleeful Buzzfeed exposé followed not long after. Mackey retired to Florida hoping to avoid further media attention, but in January 2021, just a few days after Biden took office, he was arrested in West Palm Beach on charges of interference in a federal election, for a Hillary Clinton meme encouraging black and Latino voters to cast their votes by text. Now, two years later, he's been convicted of voter suppression and faces years in jail.

Mackey's real crime was helping make the unthinkable – a Trump victory – happen. For this he had to be punished by the regime, just as Alex Jones, Steve Bannon and Roger Stone also had to be punished. What the Mackey case makes clear, and what Granza completely misses, is that anonymous posting is a key tool of political organisation on the right, one that has the power to influence, and perhaps even sway, elections. People are not posting anonymously just to pursue a career as a writer from an unusual angle, or simply to vent their frustrations about men with willies being allowed to enter women's toilets; this is not just a "culture war". At issue is the narrowing possibility of real political change, something Trump's victory genuinely represented, even if the man himself has so far failed to live up to his promise. This is why internet anonymity, in its best and worst aspects, matters and why the regime is so desperate to do away with it. Douglass Mackey is a stand-in for you, if you hadn't guessed already.

To me at least, Mark Granza's overriding concern with prestige, with the justification of anonymity solely as a pipeline to advancement in the conventional world of writing and politics, is nothing more than a reflection of his own personal aims in our sphere. He is, by his own account, an entryist, and his newfound friendship with Rod Dreher, a man who has repeatedly smeared and doxxed anonymous posters, should give us all pause for thought.

Anonymity doesn't matter only when it serves as a staging post for a career as a facephag personality on the right. In fact, when that's all it serves to do, it doesn't matter a damn, since it doesn't really change anything at all. The distinctive contribution of anons, high and low, big and small, is to say the things the regime doesn't want us to say, to break the hold of our ridiculous captured media and intellectual elites, whose venality and subservience would shame even the lowest form of communist kakocracy.

You either defend the anons – *all of us* – or you defend none of us. It's that simple. But it helps if you actually understand what we're doing, and genuinely care, in the first place. ◼

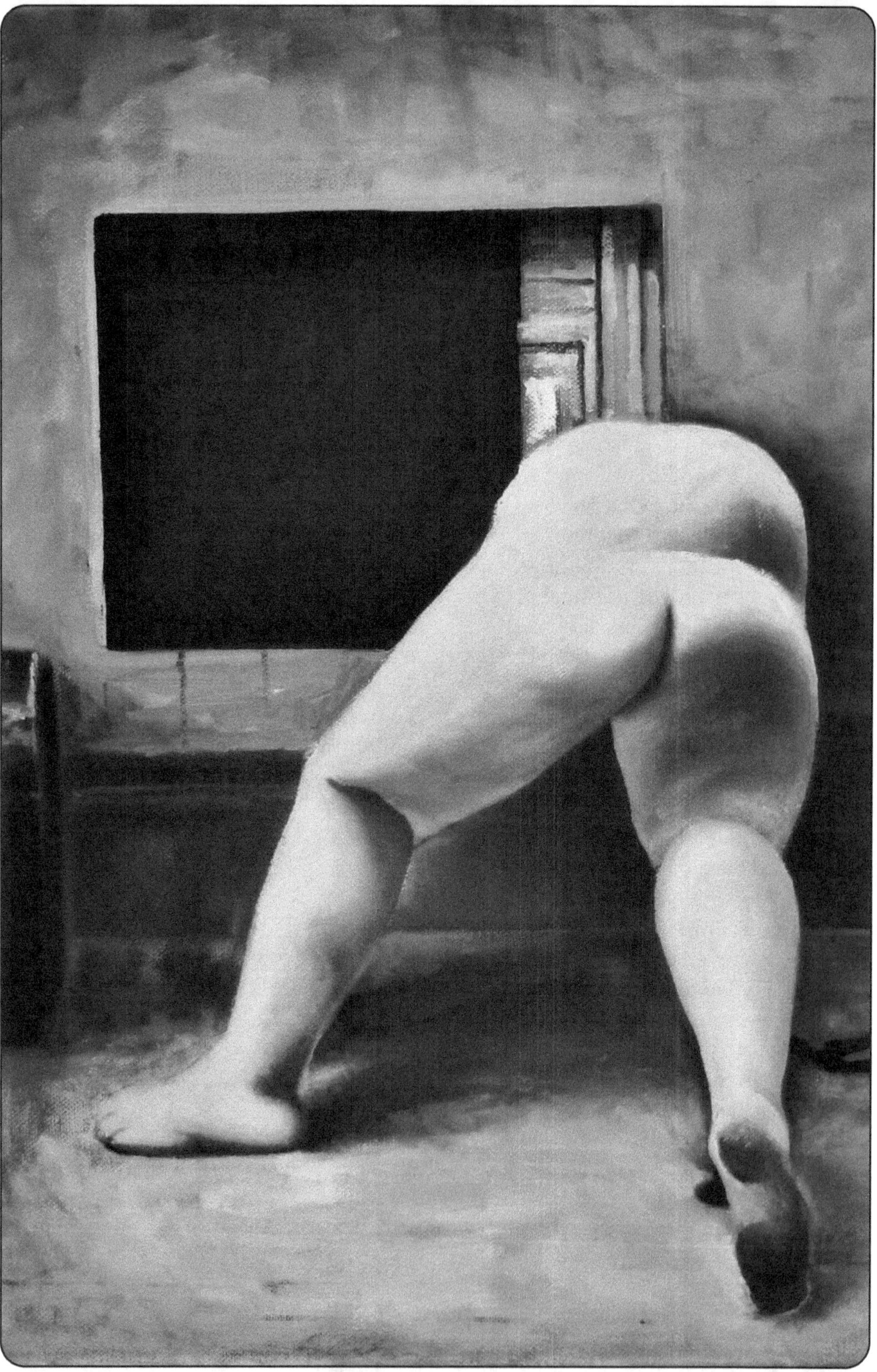

AN UNCANNY NIGHTMARE

art essay by ALEXANDER ADAMS

In his latest series of images, Alexander Adams uses AI to produce uncanny scenes that challenge us to confront the power of normality

In my previous article, I wrote about my Square Paintings, nudes in contemporary settings. The paintings illustrated here are the Uncanny Paintings, again in the square format but this time the subject matter is not nudity and eroticism, but absurdity and a nightmarish mood. Semi-human personages inhabit worlds that are familiar to ours but distorted. The absence of colour gives the scenes a 1940s atmosphere. As in my other earlier paintings, some faces are obscured. A blurred-faced woman sits on the ground in front of a Modernist housing block or industrial building. A strange beak-nosed weakling reaches for a bottle on a window sill. A beautiful headless woman reaches upwards in a curtained room, her hands turned into the predatory claws of a praying mantis.

The Uncanny Paintings came about because to explore the territory of the nightmare I had to construct disturbing imagery. I wanted to do it in a way that used AI, which would incorporate my mistrust of that technology. For me, AI is a troubling presence – a nightmare in itself. The program's lack of sentience combined with its apparent ability to discern (but not discriminate) presents a ghastly mélange of human qualities without human intelligence or agency. Like many artists, I seek new boundaries – to explore new territory. This reveals the weakness of all neophiles (lovers of the new), namely, accepting innovations that may prove misleading, harmful or

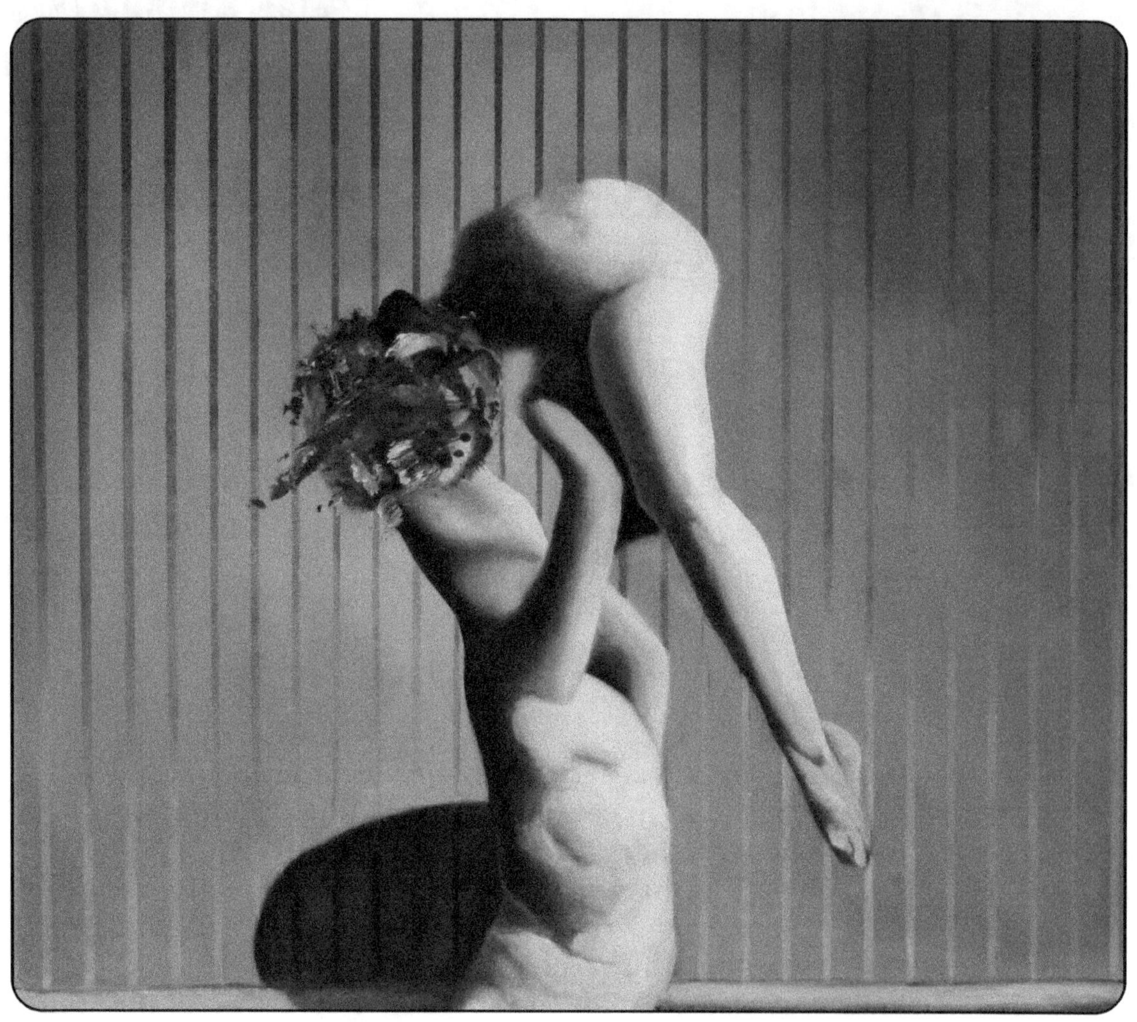

ruinous. I keep myself in check by attempting to limit innovations to those that do not depart from perennial truths: that we are emotional spiritual beings; we strive for beauty and transcendence, especially in art; we err towards sin and weakness and must combat this through mindfulness, emulation and social pressure; suffering and failure are the lot of all men; we should preserve, respect and transmit the values of our forebears but we cannot ignore the material situation we find ourselves in.

Powerful art derives most forcefully from our experiences. In creating new art which speaks about the truths of our lives, we cannot return to the classically garbed figure in an idyllic landscape, however much we might like to. Yes, such clothes can be recreated and such landscapes still exist, but is this a reflection of even our best efforts at living? Is it even within our lived experiences? Such ways of living are so distant from us that they are fantasy. As long as we are in thrall to fantasy and work towards an impossible aim, we allow the enemies of perennial truths (who are themselves utopians, albeit materialist utopians) to gain ground on us.

I put prompts into the Stable Diffusion online image-generation engine and examined the results.

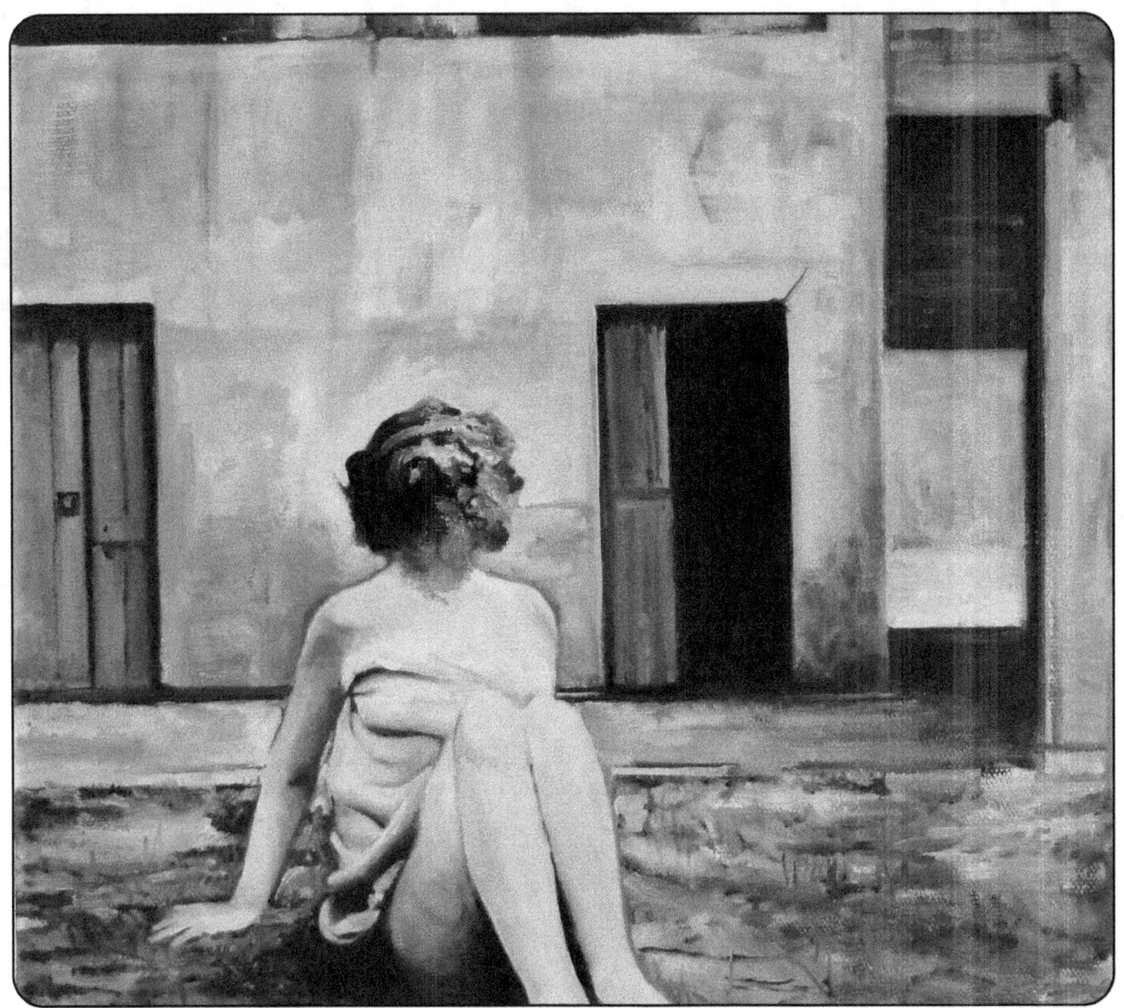

About 80% of the images produced were of little value – too jumbled, banal, visually busy, difficult to understand and lacking in visual qualities to be worthy of consideration. I printed out the few that had potential, then painted the best, making changes necessary. That meant sometimes removing extraneous elements, simplifying the space or making aspects more coherent – even if that did not mean making them more logical.

Now, as an associate and supporter of creative dissidents and dissenters on the cultural right, I lay myself open to criticism by using these methods. Those who consider themselves traditionalists and classical artists are hostile to the use of technology in artistic production, especially employing computer-derived imagery. I have no defence against such criticism other than saying that as some artists use the found image of the landscape view or adapt existing subjects (such as arranging a model or objects in a still-life), so I have also done with these AI images. The discrimination that was deployed to guide the AI program and to sort through the mass of resultant pictures was purely my own. It is down to others to decide if the Uncanny Paintings are worthwhile or a step too far.

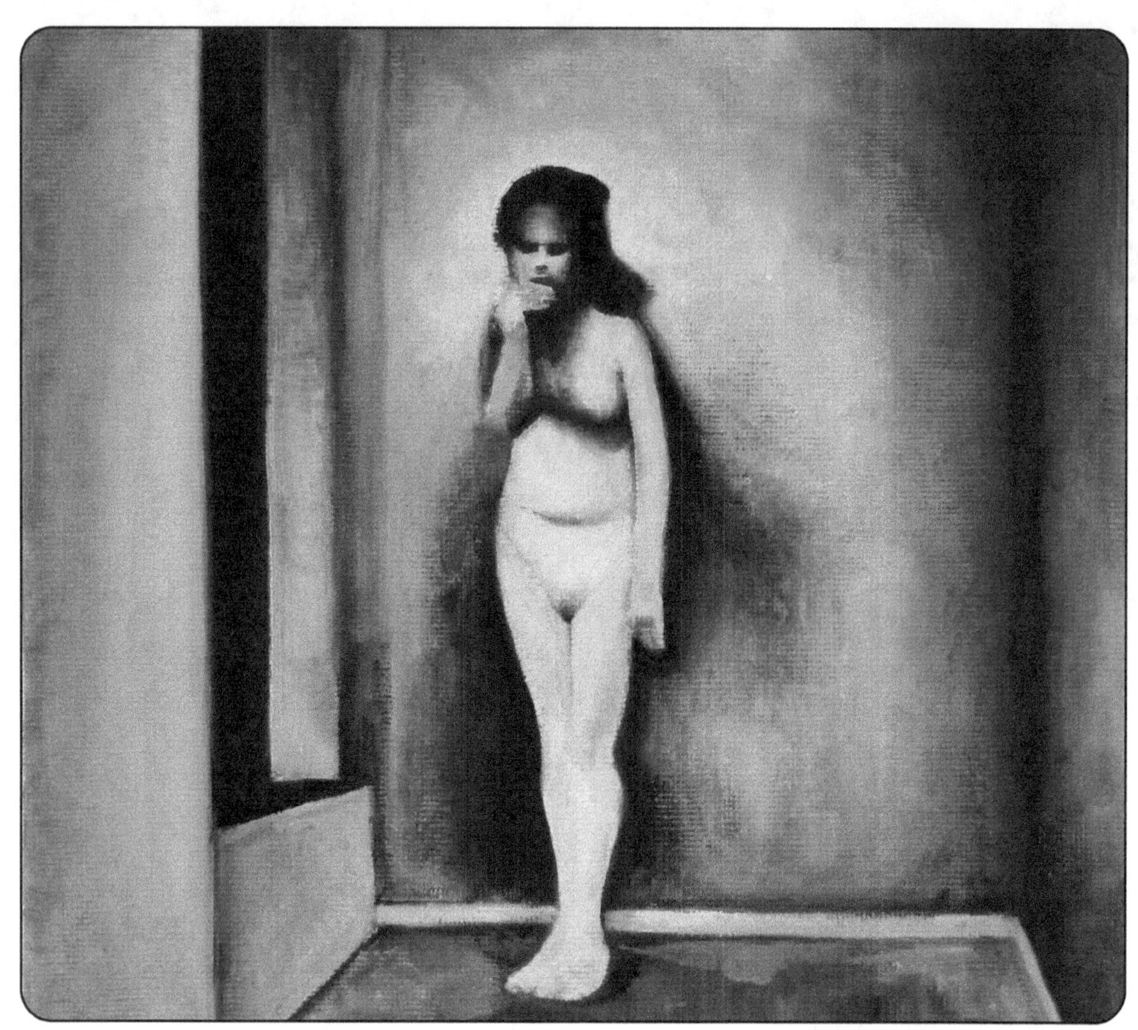

"I RECORD IMAGES THAT MOVE ME DEEPLY WITH THEIR BEAUTY, UGLINESS, STRANGENESS OR SUBLIME QUALITIES, REGARDLESS OF THE ORIGIN"

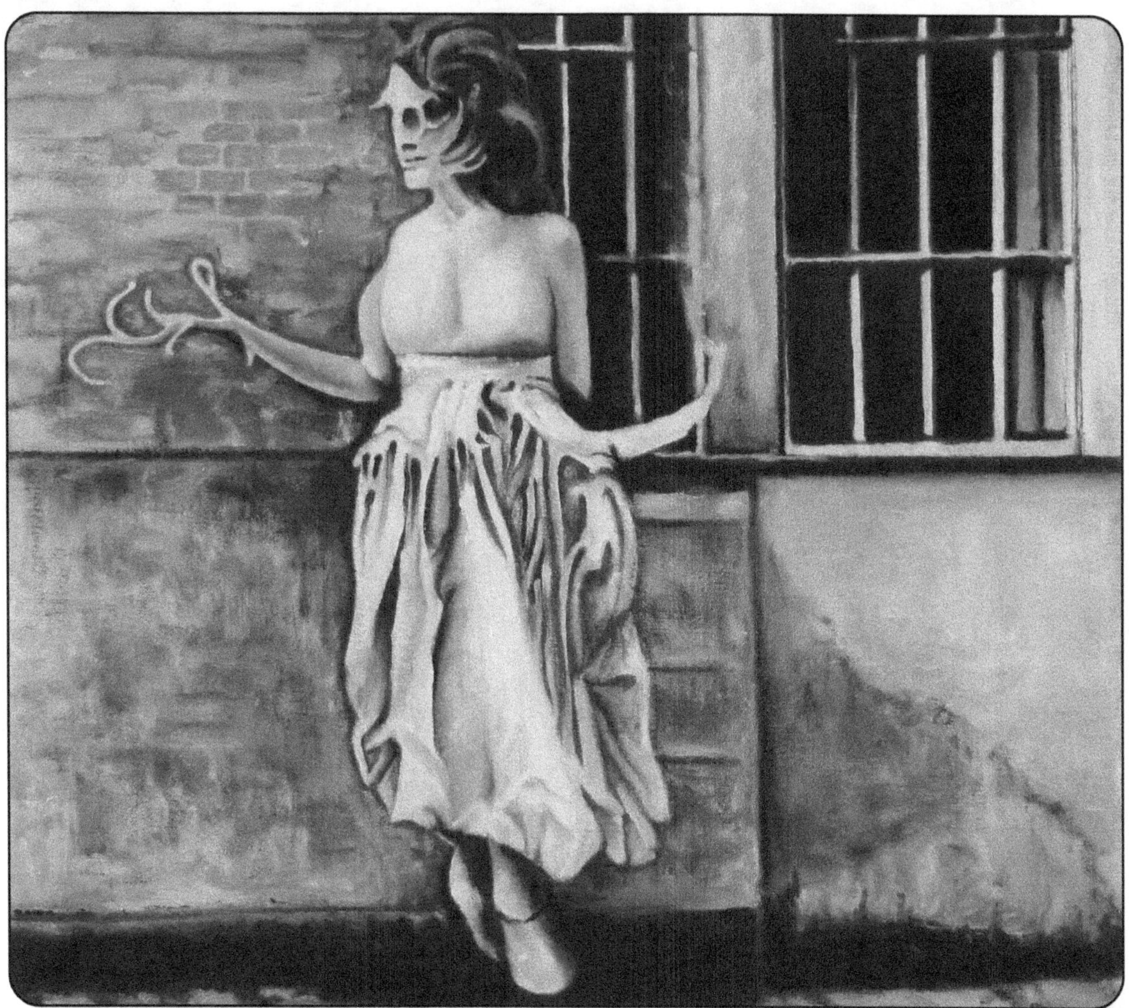

I am in search of images that are powerful; I record images that move me deeply with their beauty, ugliness, strangeness or sublime qualities, regardless of the origin. Those aspects I found in the AI images. I responded to the sources and made paintings and others have reacted strongly to their oddness.

As set out in a recent statement of principles with a group of dissenting artists I am part of, I assert the legitimacy of any means (technological, material, stylistic) to achieve successful pursuit of the beautiful, strange, foul, startling and impressive in artistic form. You may find these images terrible – I do too – but if your psyche spasms in their presence, then they have real power. If you choose to look away, no one would blame you. I ask that you consider why the images seem repellent and consider why images of Hell have inspired artists from the Gothic and Bosch up to Dalí and Beksinski. Perhaps part of the human situation is an obsession with our darkest fears. Only by seeing and understanding can we overcome fear or maybe (when facing the horror) we should step back, full of sacred fear.

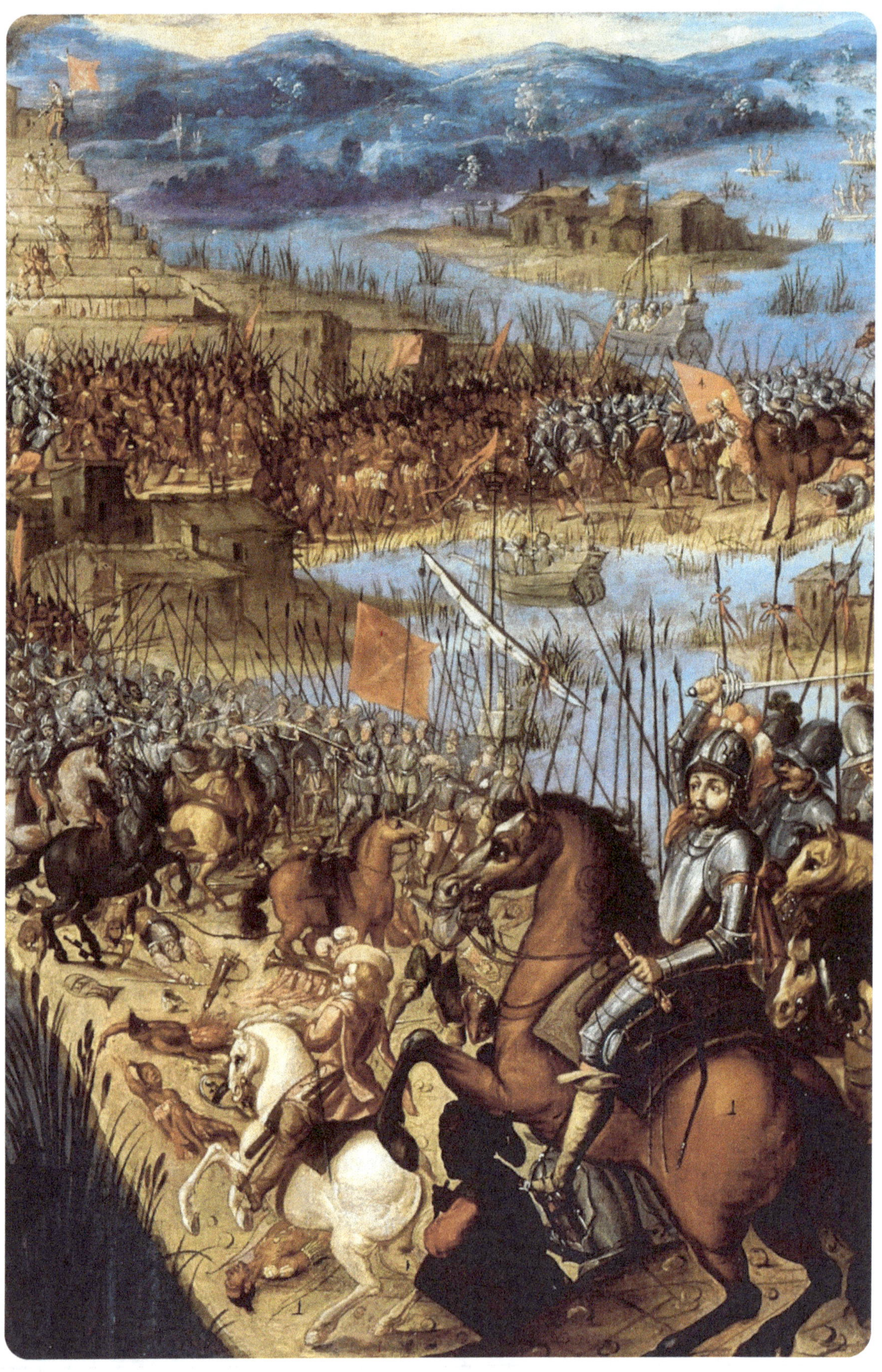

THE ENDLESS FRONTIER

essay by ALARIC THE BARBARIAN

Don't believe the doomsayers: there is always opportunity for adventure. You only have to look in the right places...

This movement – the subculture pioneered on Twitter, in this magazine, and in quiet groups around the world – is difficult to define. Whatever it is, though, it is certainly a movement to some degree characterized by historicism.

The West today has been unmoored from centuries of tradition, culture, and moral developments. We have been set adrift in a post-modern technoscape, one which is collapsing under the weight of its own ridiculous contradictions. The result is post-modernity – clown world, stuck culture, the Longhouse. A world not just lacking order and reason, but built in direct opposition to the very concept. Men are demonized, neutered. Those who built our world are slandered as a daily humiliation ritual.

As a result, many – myself included – look to history for inspiration, parallels, and guides to power and redemption. We find exemplars of greatness in Achilles, Charlemagne, Washington, Jünger, and many more. However, drawing a direct parallel to our current plight is nearly impossible. A few eras are commonly invoked, though imperfectly. The fall of Rome offers many analogues, but doesn't quite fit; the Weimar Republic is obviously apt; and in many ways the world today resembles the Balkan region prior to its collapse in the 1990s, though even this comparison is strained.

More importantly, these historical periods offer very little in

"THE FRONTIER SOUGHT BY THE LIKES OF CORTES, PIZARRO, AND THOUSANDS MORE WOULD HAVE SEEMED UNREACHABLE, EVEN FANTASTICAL IN THEIR EARLY YOUTH"

the way of hope, or even constructive insight. Rome fell as an inevitable conclusion of centuries of deracination and overextension. The Weimar Republic was addressed by a radical regime which nonetheless collapsed. The Balkans are still impoverished and violent today. All popular historic parallels end in destruction, loss, decay. But it doesn't have to be like this.

Here, I aim to offer a decidedly less well-known parallel, which perhaps offers a more helpful message. There has been a culture which faced total annihilation, yet triumphed against overwhelming odds. This same culture then narrowly averted a fade into domesticity and irrelevance via meritocracy, daring, and force of will, enjoying centuries of wealth and prominence as a result.

That culture was medieval Spain, and its redemption is the story of the conquistadors.

If you were educated in an American public school, your image of the conquistadors is likely negative. Since Howard Zinn began the propaganda campaign against the discoverers and tamers of the New World in 1980, Spanish explorers in particular have been depicted as monstrously evil, and stupid to the point of banality.

In reality, the men who discovered and conquered Central and South America were exemplars of vitality, men of a more ancient variety who regularly beat impossible odds in the name of god, glory and gold. The propaganda effort to defame the conquistadors of the 15th and 16th centuries often tends to obscure the details of their expeditions, as well as the milieu from which they arose. This milieu is perhaps just as important as their stories in themselves, and no writing on the conquistadors would be complete without a discussion of their forefathers: the hidalgos, pioneers and soldiers of the Reconquista.

From the invasion of Iberia in 711 by Muslim forces to the Spanish victory at Grenada in 1492, the peoples of the Iberian peninsula were engaged in a life-and-death struggle against Islamic rule of the region. Various kingdoms and peoples engaged in this centuries-long struggle, a civilizational clash between Christianity and Islam which claimed thousands of lives across generations on both sides. As this conflict raged, a caste of knightly nobility rose on the Christian side: the hidalgos, mounted warriors who entered the knighthood by ancestry or service. They fought for the Spanish crown, as well as for personal wealth. Areas reclaimed from Muslim forces could be granted to them as *encomienda*, a system of rewarding personal valor with

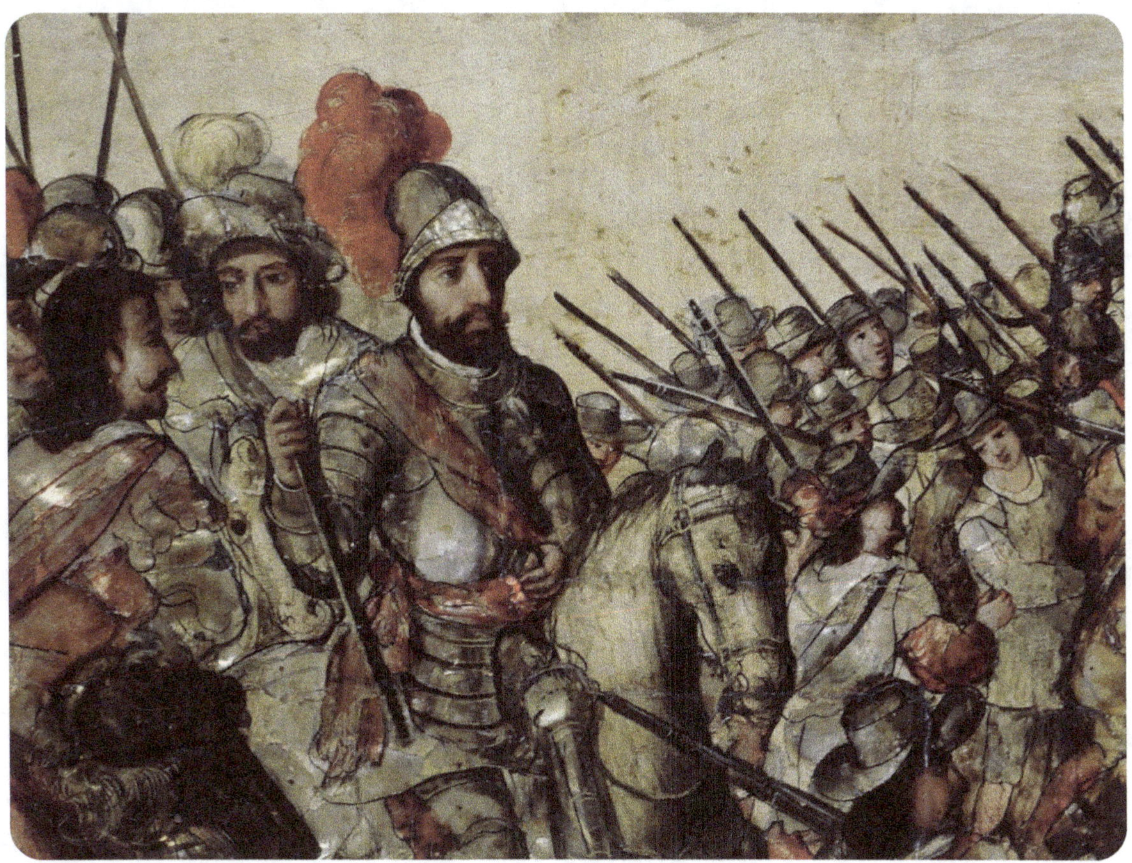

land and labor which later became the blueprint for Spanish expansion in the New World.

Additionally, simple footsoldiers participating in the Reconquista could expect financial rewards for their service, and perhaps afford entry into this knightly class after years of outstanding service. Thus, the bloody frontier between Spain and Islamic-controlled regions became a potent place for meritocracy in medieval Spanish culture, where young men could test themselves in battle and perhaps attain command, wealth, and glory.

Over the course of this 700-year conflict, Spain evolved culturally and militarily to counter the Moorish threat. A strong frontiersman ethos took hold, and a deeply Catholic martial spirit became a defining characteristic of the Spanish people. The Spanish in many ways became an expeditionary culture, as the war with the Moors ebbed and flowed over the centuries.

By the mid-15th century, this frontier was beginning to close. After seven centuries of brutal back-and-forth conflict, the Iberian peninsula was almost entirely controlled by Spain, with the exception of a limited region surrounding Grenada. The frontier was no longer as lucrative as it had been in the 13th-14th centuries, and a number of hidalgos fell into poverty or at least idleness. Many applied their martial talents as mercenaries in Italy or elsewhere – though these conflicts were not nearly as profitable as the Moorish frontier had once been.

The true crisis came with the sons

of these men, who truly lacked the opportunity once presented to their fathers, especially after Granada fell, at last, in 1492. The Moorish frontier was no longer the place to test oneself for wealth and honor, and their fathers – born-and-raised fighting men – had little advice for their sons as to how to navigate a world without a frontier. Hernan Cortes was one of these young men, with a surplus of martial will and a deficit of opportunity. Instead of sending him to the frontlines, his parents opted to send him to the city for legal training, entering him into what seemed to be the most lucrative environment in a new era of Spain – one defined by clerks, lawyers, finances.

Of course, Cortes had little care for such a career, and we know where he ended up instead. But is this story not a parallel to many struggles today? Out-of-touch parents offering advice after having grown up in an entirely different world, their sons floundering due to a lack of the same opportunities presented to their parents. An economy faced with lowering standards, in a nation seemingly unmoored from its core ethos. No lucrative frontier of meritocracy for ambitious young men. The desire for martial conquest and glory sublimated into paperwork, banality, domesticity. Vitality crushed under the weight of pure mundaneness.

Francisco Pizarro is perhaps the most extreme example of this situation. As the bastard son of infantry colonel Gonzalo Pizarro, he was raised in poverty without the expectation of any inheritance or title. His mother was a peasant, and thus he spent the first thirty-odd years of his life as a simple swineherd for his father's pigs. It was only in the wild, unforgivingly meritocratic New World that he would be able to demonstrate his personal valor and talent for command.

The frontier sought by the likes of Cortes, Pizarro, and thousands more would have seemed unreachable, even fantastical in their early youth. Spain had built a caste of frontiersmen which, with the reconquest of Granada in 1492, had lost their frontier. In that same year, however, the Spanish court decided to finance an absurd risk in the expedition of Christopher Columbus, allegedly to find a shorter route to China.

Funding Columbus' expedition was truly a "moonshot" effort. In yet another parallel to our situation today, Spain was rapidly losing military and economic power to a more manoeuvrable nation: Portugal. As the first and preeminent investor in sailing technology and exploration, the Portuguese had a grip on international trade, particularly in resource-rich West Africa and, after Bartolomeu Dias' expedition around the Cape of Good Hope in 1448, India. Spain had entered the maritime race late and without any of the built-up expertise of the Portuguese. The Spanish economic situation was dire, by comparison.

So, when Columbus came to the Spanish court with a ludicrous proposal, based on what was clearly bunk science (namely the claim that Earth was half its known size), the Spanish court was willing to entertain him for longer than the Portuguese. Sensing that he was hiding something, they continued to deliberate over the proposal for a full two years. A western trade route to China was clearly impossible – but based on Columbus' terms, it seemed that he may have been onto something far more valuable. Something he was unwilling to disclose, but willing to bet his life on.

When Columbus threatened to take the idea to France, going as far as to ride a donkey out of Spain, Ferdinand and Isabella capitulated, sending a messenger to inform him that the voyage would be funded. A few months later, in October 1492 – only nine months after Granada had been retaken, officially ending the Reconquista – Columbus landed in the New World.

With the first steps taken on that new land, the frontier had opened for the Spanish people once again, setting the stage for the incredible victories of the conquistadors. The historian Samuel Eliot Morison describes the gravity of the moment well:

"Other discoveries there have been more spectacular than that of this small, flat sandy island that rides out ahead of the American continent, breasting the trade winds. But it was there that the Ocean for the first time "loosed the chains of things" as Seneca had prophesied, gave up the secret that had baffled Europeans since they began to inquire what lay beyond the western horizon's rim. Stranger people than the gentle Tainos, more exotic plants than the green verdure of Guanahani have been discovered, even by the Portuguese before Columbus; but the discovery of Africa was but an unfolding of a continent already glimpsed, whilst San Salvador, rising from the sea at the end of a thirty-three-day westward sail, was a clean break with past experience."

This was a world-shifting moment, something that would have been impossible to anticipate by any contemporary observer. An entire new continent, populated and resource-rich, seemingly open to be claimed by Spain alone. All it took was one man unwilling to be told no, with a vision far greater than that of his kinsmen. Just when it seemed that the frontier was closed, that no untamed fringe of civilization would be open for enterprising men – Columbus set foot on an entirely untouched *continent*.

Today, a common lament in certain corners is the lack of a true frontier. I imagine that the same lament would have been heard among young descendants of the hidalgo in 1492. However, all it took was one true visionary genius to change this – opening a frontier on a scale incomprehensible to previous generations.

But this is not all. The conquests undertaken by the Spanish were unique – they attained total control, total ownership over the lands they explored. New Spain was truly New Spain: a Catholic land entirely governed by the Spanish crown. Unlike French or early British expeditions to North America, Spain mobilized a massive number of fighting men to the New World, all with conquest and glory on their minds – not mere trade or exile. The frontiersman ethos of the Reconquista was turned across the Atlantic, to the exotic and dangerous lands of the Aztec and Inca Empires.

Among these men were a few of a certain caliber, who distinguished themselves above the rest. The explorers Enciso, Balboa, and de Soto; the warriors Pedro de Alvarado and Diego de Almagro; and the leader-conquerors Hernan Cortes and Francisco Pizarro; among many more. The vast frontier of the Americas selected for a certain sort of individual, one whose example may be worth studying today. All of these men rose from the same set of circumstances that concern young men today: economic uncertainty, stifling domesticity, and the lack of a true frontier. And yet they rose to the occasion of a new opportunity, inscribing their names in history for centuries to come.

Among them, particularly Cortes and Pizarro, there are a few common traits worth examining. The first and most outstanding is a trait seen often among the great men of history: an incredible personal magnetism. People rallied around them almost as a matter of course, and they seemed to inspire men to offer their sword.

For Cortes, this personal magnetism was in large part due to his oratory, rhetorical skill, and theatrical flair. He understood how to give a speech that would rally ambitious men to his side. Nothing exemplifies this better than Cortes' initial recruitment for his expedition to Mexico, an unknown land which had claimed the lives of two prior expeditions. Soon after issuing Cortes' charter, the Governor of New Spain – Diego Velazquez – revoked it due to personal issues with the explorer. Knowing Cortes' strong will, he sent men to reign him in and if necessary, perform an arrest.

Knowing that he had limited time, Cortes took a hurried tour around taverns and meeting-places, rallying six ships and 300 fully-equipped men in less than a month. The speeches he gave to these men are lost to history, but one must imagine that they rival those given to the ten thousand Greeks in the Anabasis. Upon landing with those men at Veracruz, he further inspired confidence and conviction by ordering their ships dismantled and burned, to remove any way out of Mexico except victory over the Aztecs.

But this is not all. Later, when Velazquez sent a 1,000-strong expedition to Mexico to arrest Cortes, he bested them in combat – and then convinced the survivors to join him. Of course, this all goes without delving into his expert navigation of native alliances and tensions, which by 1521 gained him over 100,000 Tlaxcala allies. The men who conquered New Spain were, above all, characters of incredibly strong will and presence – and Cortes was the strongest and had the greatest presence of them all.

As for Pizarro, exactly how he inspired this magnetism is not well-documented, but in large part it seems to have been due to his unceasing drive, decisiveness, and unwillingness to accept no for an answer. In 1526, after multiple failed expeditions south of Spanish territory, he and his men had once again run into hostile natives and were out of supplies. Knowing that the governor of Panama would not sanction any further exploration upon his return, Pizarro chose to stay on an unpopulated island and wait for a ship to return to his rescue, so that he could take it and continue exploring.

It was there, at Isla de Gallo, that he gave his famous speech in opposition to his comrades' desire to return home: "There lies Peru with its riches; Here, Panama and its poverty. Choose, each man, what best becomes a brave Castilian. For my part, I go to the south." It inspired thirteen men to stay with him on that island, waiting seven months for his fellow conquistadors Almagro and de Luque to return. Later, once his expedition to the interior of Peru began, he issued similarly terse and stoic proclamations. One report holds that after one of his men was caught hoarding gold, he ordered that man's share distributed among the others, and then, since he could never expect someone to work without pay, that he be executed. Later, at Cajamarca, this decisiveness, vigor, and force of will would gain him and his men an empire. The plot to kidnap Atahualpa from amidst his men was, on its face, absurd – and yet, Pizarro's men followed his lead and did not desert or rout.

They won the day without taking a single casualty, and conquered the entirety of Peru in the process.

However, this force of character and rhetorical skill cannot be invoked without mentioning the open defiance of authority shared by both conquerors. When Cortes left for Mexico in 1519, it was an act of open mutiny against the leader of New Spain. And yet, with no one to physically stop him and the resources at his disposal rather than the governor's, he went ahead anyway. This complete disregard for any authority besides his own is the why Cortes conquered Mexico, and was a large part of the reason that his men followed him so adamantly.

Pizarro first defied his superiors by continuing the expedition after being picked up from Isla de Gallo, much to Governor Pedro de los Rios's chagrin. Later, when he appealed directly to the Spanish court for a commission to conquer Peru, he was given very specific terms in the *Capitulacion de Toledo*, signed by Queen Isabel herself: he was to raise 150 equipped men before leaving for the New World, where he could recruit another 100. However, after recruiting as many of his relatives and friends as possible, he failed to meet the number, and openly defied the Spanish crown by sailing secretly – under cover of darkness – away from Castille. In both cases, force of will and individual power overrode the authorities supposed to restrain these men; and in both cases, they were able to succeed on their own terms.

The third quality common to these men, as well as their subordinates and the thousands of others who built the Spanish New World, is a deep sense of religious zeal. Today, this is perhaps a controversial claim to make about the conquistadors. They have been stereotyped as gold-hungry buffoons wearing their religion as a mere decoration. However, a proper study of their own writings completely dispels this propagandized notion. From Cortes and Pizarro to their lieutenants and down to their lowest servants, the exploration and conquest of the Spanish New World was character-

HERODOTEAN FIRE
BY LYCURGUS

ized by an incredible dedication to the Christian faith, on a level almost incomprehensible today.

These men saw themselves as having been animated to conquest by God himself, to do His will in a demonic land characterized by human sacrifice and bloodlust. They ventured into a true heart of darkness – in the Andes, the Amazon, or in the jungles and marshes of the Yucatan. And after their conquests were secured, they worked to proselytize to the natives, making a genuine effort to convert as many as possible – an effort which shaped South America into one of the world's most strongly Catholic regions to this day.

But I am not here to argue the Christianity of the conquistadors, only to see what can be drawn from their example. In this case, their religious zeal led to a clarity of purpose which is almost impossible to replicate today. Their writings show no self-consciousness, no questioning, no weakness of will; only dedication, conviction, drive. They had a mission and were dedicated to it above all else: conquer the New World in the name of Christ and the Spanish crown. And they had no doubt about their justification: *God wills it.* This level of assuredness should serve as inspiration today, in a world so defined by noncommittal thinking and existential doubt. Of course, such dedication can only be built upon a foundation of physical strength and vitality – which the conquistadors certainly possessed.

The frontier is never closed, even when it seems like the world is entirely tamed and owned. And if you can find that frontier, there is no limit to what can be accomplished with conviction, character, and sheer force of will. The stories of the conquistadors still hold untold wisdom, especially for those who feel stifled by the modern world.

I believe that the future will be defined not by preachers of weakness and humility – but by unstoppable men like Christopher Columbus, Hernan Cortes, and Francisco Pizarro. *God wills it.* ◼

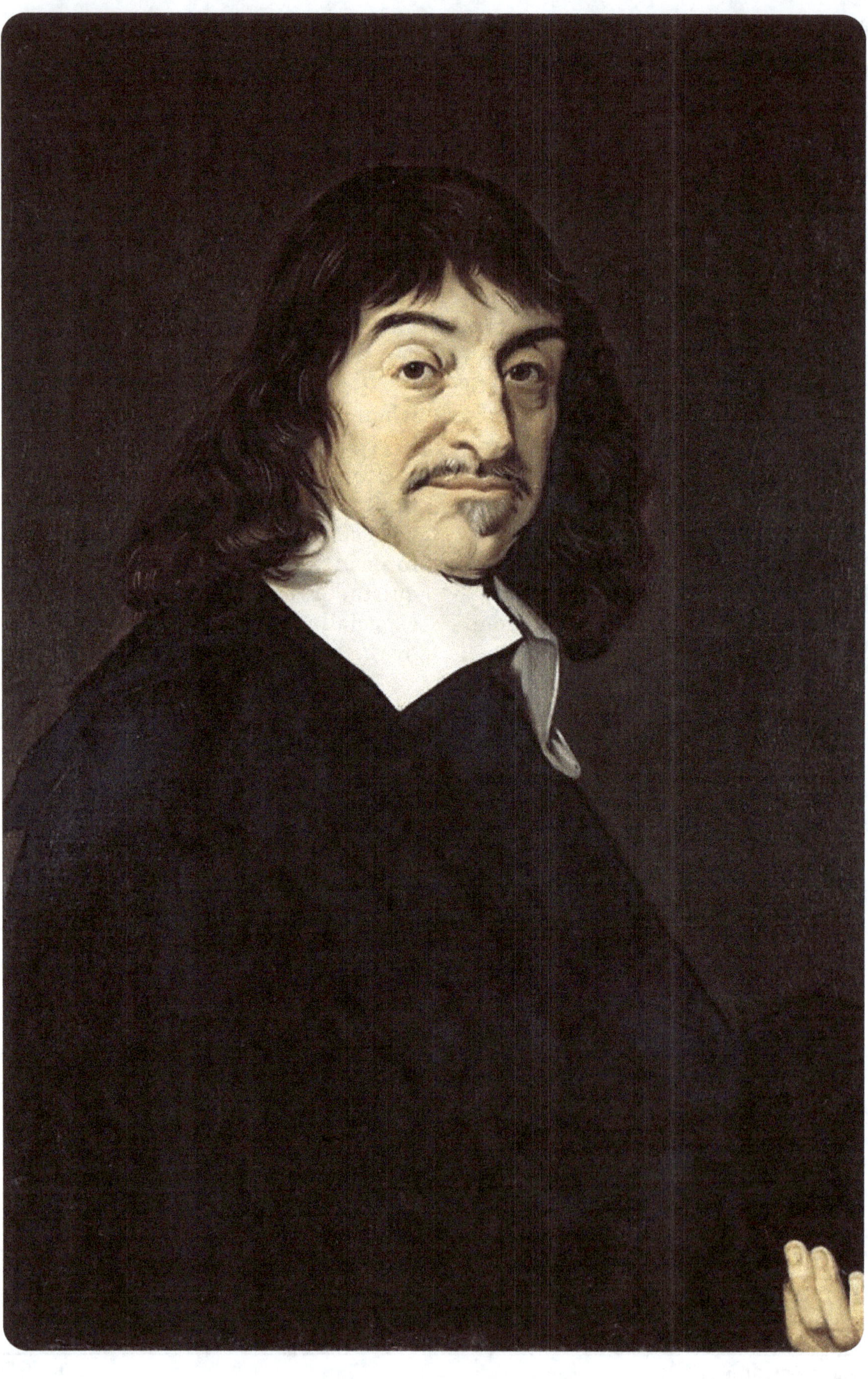

THE DECLINE OF INTUITION

essay by TÓLMA

What happens when thought turns against life and becomes an enemy to it? Descartes, supposedly an arch-rationalist, knew all too well...

I. Difficult modernity

To contemporary readers, Descartes is most known as the philosopher who separated mind from body and replaced traditional philosophy with a new scientific method. As such, his name itself has come to stand for all that we deem wrong with the modern world —man's separation from nature and the consequent environmental destruction, the failures of allopathic science-based medicine, and a world void of poetry. As much as there might be a real line of development between these wrongs and revolutionary thinkers such as Descartes, the complete story of philosophical modernity's founder is much more complex, and much more beautiful.

It is true, Descartes separated soul from body and came to see man and nature as nothing more than machines. But we learn absolutely nothing if we do not ask why Descartes did so in the first place, if we do not ask after the spirit of this man that thought it necessary to re-think everything we hold dear and true. Why understand the body as a machine? So we can further our knowledge of medicine and live more healthy and powerful lives, and so we can stop feeling guilty for our sad passions, when they might just be caused by bodily indigestion due to a bad diet. And why should we understand the soul as indubitably certain in its separation from the body? So that, whatever might happen and however confused the world might get, we always have a stronghold against deception. You can deceive me, and I can even deceive myself, but I still am; at least this is certain.

And *even if* no one today can honestly believe in the key tenets of Cartesianism, the spirit of Descartes' philosophy can still inspire us. This spirit is one of creativity, confidence, and a unique desire for philosophy to be in the service of life. That is, for Descartes, philosophy should serve to give us clear and distinct knowledge so we can better guide our actions and "walk confidently through this life."

Looking around at the philosophy of his time, Descartes noticed something peculiar. Philosophy should bring us closer to truth and enhance our lives. Yet, it seems that the more philosophers think, the more confused they become. The more they question, the less confident they get, and the less capable of action they become. Every idiot on the streets knows he exists, but the philosophers question whether they even exist, and they even question the value of existence. In the end, who is it that deserves to be called a lover of wisdom?

Hence Descartes' question: why does thought turn against the thinker, why does it make us weaker and more confused, when it should serve to make us stronger and wiser? And, his project: the construction of simple truths clear and evident by grace of pure intuition, so that thought can stop being an enemy to life, and regain its rightful place as life's most powerful ally.

II. Confidence as first philosophy

In Descartes' dialogue, *The Search for Truth by Means of the Natural Light*, we witness three men having a philosophical discussion. There is Polyander, a lay-
man who served his life in the army and never enjoyed any higher education. We have Epistemon, a respected philosopher at the schools, deeply familiar with the tradition and the intricacies of scholastic philosophy. Finally, there is Eudoxus, representing Descartes himself. Like Epistemon, Eudoxus is a philosopher, but of an entirely different kind. He too studied at the schools, but after a while, he realized that he would be better off doing philosophy in a new manner, away from the academic way of doing things:

"I do not wish to examine what others have examined or ignored. I am satisfied in remarking that even if all the knowledge that one could desire were to be contained in books, the good in them would be intermingled with so many useless things, and scattered confusedly throughout such a massive pile of tomes, that we would need more time for reading them than we have in this life, and more spirit for determining what is useful, than we would need for coming up with it ourselves."

And so, Eudoxus left the schools to travel the world and think for himself. He is the private thinker as opposed to the university philosopher. In our dialogue, Polyander comes to the two philosophers because he would like to know a thing or two about philosophy, and the result is Eudoxus and Epistemon fighting over the correct method to instruct him. Moreover, they differ in their opinions on whether Polyander is even capable of learning much in the first place. According to Epistemon, Polyander should not hope for too much, for it takes a lifetime of being occupied with the most important texts of phi-

"PHILOSOPHY SHOULD BRING US CLOSER TO TRUTH AND ENHANCE OUR LIVES. YET, IT SEEMS THAT THE MORE PHILOSOPHERS THINK, THE MORE CONFUSED THEY BECOME"

losophy, and even then,

"The desire for knowledge, common to all men, is like an illness which cannot be cured, for curiosity grows with learning."

And so he tries to dissuade Polyander: if I as a great philosopher can't even attain the truth, then you certainly can't. Epistemon goes on to hammer away further at Polyander's confidence. The layman, at first happy to meet a few philosophers and ready to learn about the nature of reality, is now overcome with shame and an acute awareness of his own inadequacies, forever distanced from the experts by his ignorance, as man is from God.

However, Eudoxus disagrees with Epistemon, and he says to Polyander: you too can attain knowledge of those things most worth knowing. All it takes is the natural light of your own reason, a bit of common sense, and the will to truly and honestly think. Granted, you started late in life, and maybe you won't have the time to read everything Aristotle or Aquinas wrote, but since when is the power of one's thought measured by what one has read? The point is not to memorize Aristotle's works, but like Aristotle to engage in an honest search for truth. And you too can do this, as long as you are willing.

What happens is a sort of conversion of the soul, where Polyander goes from a layman ashamed of his own ignorance, convinced he will never know anything, to a man confident in his abilities to know the truth and act on it. This is why we can say that with Descartes, confidence is first philosophy. For before one can hope to know anything, one needs the confidence to truly think. This is all that "enlightenment" means.

As Kant thinks about the abstract transcendental conditions required for knowledge, Descartes thinks about the real existential conditions for thought. What type of man will attain the fruits of philosophy? The man who is willing to think, whose confidence hasn't been crushed by education, and who doesn't need the assistance of common opinion. This is Descartes' idea, naive perhaps, but honest.

III. The problem of intuition (so intelligent they even doubt themselves)

At a crucial point in *The Search for Truth*, Eudoxus leads Polyander to the famous Cartesian proof: "I think, (and therefore) I am." Polyander is asked to doubt everything he can possibly doubt, and he soon realizes that if he does so, there is one thing he cannot doubt: the fact that he is doubting. And what is doubting? Well, a type of thinking. And if it is certain that I am thinking, then at least I know that I exist as a thinking thing. I might not know anything else about myself for the moment, but at least I know that I am a thinking thing. And so Polyander realizes that even if as an uncultured layman he doesn't know anything, he at least knows that he exists. It might not be much, but it is in any case more than those contemporary philosophers and scientists who go on and on about 'the self' not existing, or who question if there even is such a thing as truth.

Having gone through the reasoning by his own powers, Polyander rejoices. He, a simple layman, has attained what since Ancient thought has always been seen as the highest type of knowledge: self-knowledge, a thought that is able to think itself. But Polyander's excitement doesn't last long, as Epistemon comes in to crush his confidence once again:

"You say you exist and that you know that you exist, because you are doubting and because you are thinking. But what doubting is, and what thinking is, do you even know this?"

Eudoxus responds:

"I don't think there has ever been anyone so stupid that they first had to learn what existence was before they could conclude and affirm that they exist. And the same goes for 'doubting' and 'thinking'."

What is at stake is whether there are things of which we can be immediately certain, purely by grace of intuition, without needing an elaborate reasoning or definition for their existence. Can certain things, like our own existence or thought, be clear to us in and by themselves? It is a question of intuition, which Epistemon seems to lack. How is it that a simple layman like Polyander has an intuition of his own existence, whereas a professional thinker like Epistemon needs a definition for existence before he can conclude that he exists? Whose thinking is more autonomous, powerful, and capable? This becomes Descartes' problem.

The idea: there is a terrible danger to philosophy. Thinking and reading so much, filling one's mind with all sorts of opinions, one can lose the ability to use one's own common sense or intuition. Moreover, one becomes so trained in argumentation and logic that one attacks even those truths so clear that they do not even need logic to stand on their feet.

In his *Principles of Philosophy*, Descartes states, "I have noticed that philosophers, in trying to explain by the rules of their logic things that are manifest by themselves, have done nothing but obscure them." Why, asks Descartes, does philosophy — that noble pursuit that should give us clear truths so we can act in this life with more confidence — turn into an incessant questioning, no longer bringing us closer to the truth, but dragging us away from it? Why do philosophers, questioning after the nature of existence, end up taking pleasure in denying their own existence? Setting out to make our lives better, philosophy ends up making life impossible.

IV. Immediate certainty

Explicitly positing himself against Descartes, Nietzsche writes:

"There are still harmless self-observers who believe in the existence of "immediate certainties," such as "I think," [...] When I dissect the process expressed in the proposition "I think,"

I get a whole set of bold claims that are difficult, perhaps impossible, to establish, —for instance, that I am the one who is thinking, that there must be something that is thinking in the first place, that thinking is an activity and the effect of a being who is considered the cause, that there is an 'I,' and finally, that it has already been determined what is meant by thinking, —that I *know* what thinking is."

What do we see here but a new Epistemon? In essence, philosophy is a sort of thinking that thinks against mere opinion, against doxa, but taking this idea to its limit, things can get quite unhinged. And from Descartes' perspective, we fall into all sorts of absurdities, such as philosophers questioning the truth of their own existence because they do not yet have a clear definition of existence. Or, like Nietzsche, attacking Descartes' proof with all sorts of questions —"What is thinking?"— even such questions already presuppose thought in the way Descartes understood it.

Thought, for Descartes, is nothing but the basic fact of awareness that accompanies any and all experience. In the second meditation, it is said that even if I can doubt everything that I see with my eyes (I might be dreaming or hallucinating), I cannot doubt the fact that I have the sensation of seeing. "*At certe videre videor*", it certainly seems to me that I see. This seeming, this basic fact of awareness that accompanies any and all experience whatsoever, this is what Descartes calls thought.

Why, then, use the word "thought"? Well, if I were to say, for example: "I walk, therefore I am," one could easily think this presupposes the existence of a body, working legs, an entire sensory apparatus, and so on. And these things can be doubted. Now, if I say: "I think I am walking, and therefore I am." It could be the case that I am dreaming and that I am not walking at all, but I still cannot doubt that I am thinking that I am walking. That it seems to me that I am walking, at least this is certain. This is all that thought means, and nothing else.

We can only see the truly radical nature of Nietzsche's questions when we accept that he is attacking even Descartes' most simple claim to certainty. Even this, that it seems to me that I am seeing, the mere fact of appearing, and that at least this is certain, not even this survives the Nietzschean moment. And today, we cannot take anything whatsoever as true on the basis of intuition or common sense. We know too much to be able to know anything at all.

No one should deny that this Nietzschean way of questioning is an interesting route for thought to go down, an absolute mad questioning, ad infinitum. Has thought ever seen such power? But one must stop to look at what it presupposes. It presupposes precisely the peculiar type of stupidity Descartes points to: questioning if you know anything about your existence, even though these very questions presuppose your existence. Questioning thought, even though this questioning itself is a type of thought. What does it lead to, when you can not take anything whatsoever as evident? What will you take as evident, if it isn't your own experience and thought?

We have to recognize that Descartes was perfectly capable of questioning his "I think" like Nietzsche would do, as is evidenced by the appearance of Epistemon. Descartes had a clear idea

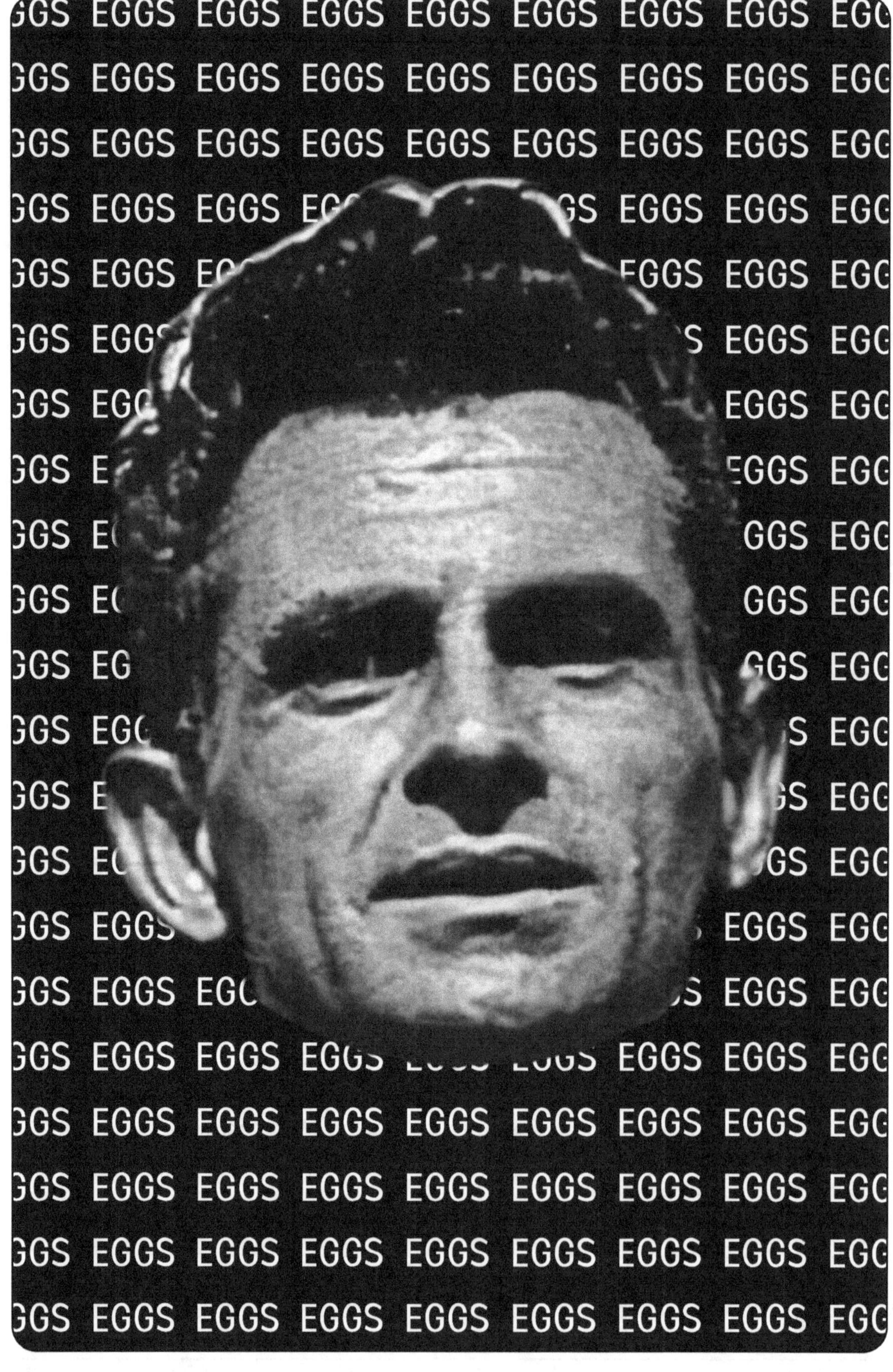

EGGS EGGS EGGS EGGS EGGS EGGS EGGS EGGS EGGS
EGGS EGGS EGGS EGGS EGGS EGGS EGGS EGGS EGGS
EGGS EGGS EGGS EGGS EGGS EGGS EGGS EGGS EGGS
EGGS EGGS EGGS EGGS EGGS EGGS EGGS EGGS EGGS
EGGS EGGS EGGS EGGS EGGS EGGS EGGS EGGS EGGS
EGGS EGGS EGGS EGGS EGGS EGGS EGGS EGGS EGGS

New Occidental Poetry

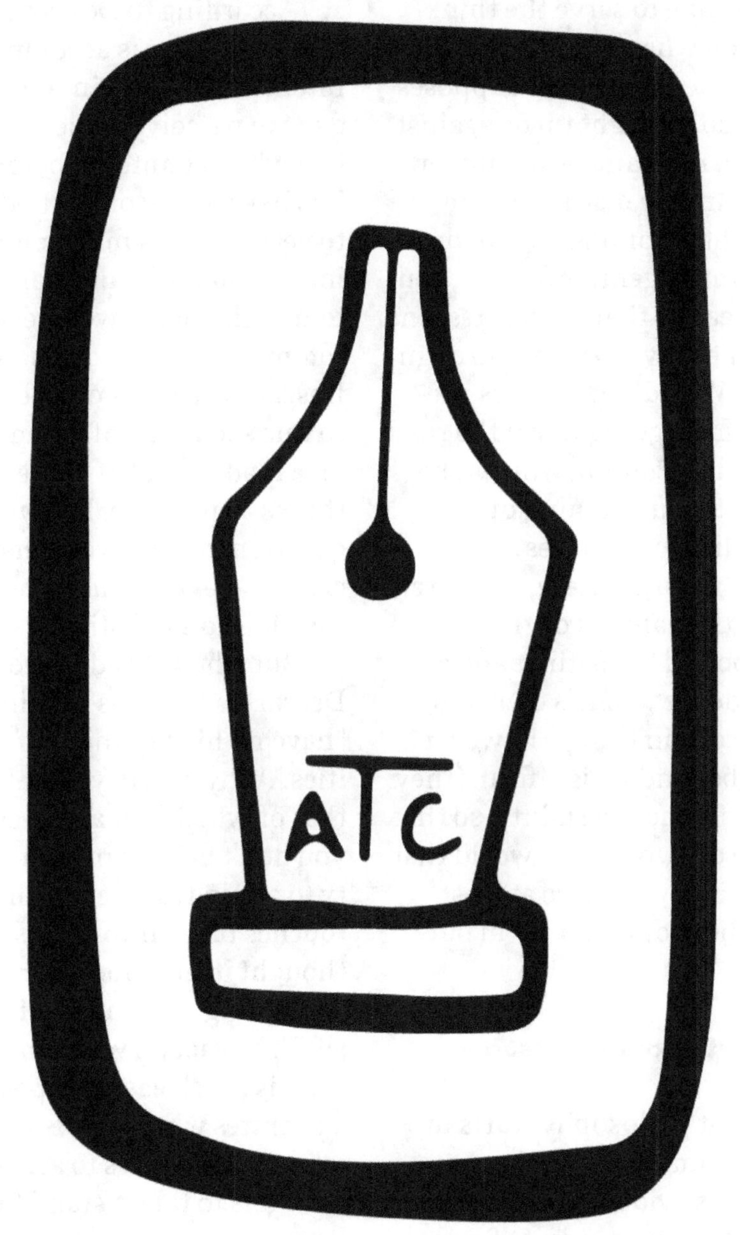

ATOPTHECLIFFS.COM

of where thought would go if it questioned even such basic intuitions, but he simply didn't want to go there. Questioning even this, for Descartes, would amount to a type of circular stupidity, a sure road to madness, and the end of thought being able to serve the thinker. You question what "I think" means, but your very questioning presupposes thought. And so, thought turns against itself, and it turns against the thinker. Like an autoimmune disease on the level of thought. I, for one, do not deem myself more intelligent, reflective, courageous, or creative than Descartes, and I take it as imperative to think through this question: Why did Descartes prevent thought from going down the road of total problematization, why did he despise this total questioning of any and all immediate certainties?

There is a "vitalism" here, a concrete awareness of the dangers of theory when not bound by instinct and a healthy confidence in one's own abilities to know certain things, however small in number and insignificant they might be. Confidence, certainty, so that even if we are drowning in a world that deceives us at every step, we at least have a stronghold of certainty in ourselves.

V. Descartes' anti-philosophy

It is said that philosophy starts in wonder, this moment in which what first appeared as evident becomes question-worthy. And since at least Socrates, philosophy has always characterized itself as an incessant questioning. It presupposes a peculiar type of madness to ask "What is Being?" or "What is thought?" Descartes agrees that philosophy starts in wonder, but it should always ensure that it escapes from wonder and arrives at truth. From question to answer, from confusion to certainty. The problem is that it is always much easier to keep wondering, than it is to act on what one knows.

According to Descartes, the sensation of wonder is accompanied by an intense excitation in the brain. In wonder, we perceive something new that we haven't encountered before. As such, it is like a stressor the body isn't used to yet, leaving a much more intense impact on the brain than merely contemplating what we already know. This intense excitation can be addictive, says Descartes. And as one becomes addicted to this sensation of wonder, one goes on a mad quest to wonder at as many things as possible. Everything must be questioned, and even what is perfectly clear and evident must be distorted to turn it into a question.

But who gets addicted to wonder? Descartes says it is usually those who "have no high opinion of their abilities." Why? Well, you only question that of which you aren't certain, and if you don't believe in your own capacity to attain truth, everything thought touches turns into a question, including thought itself. Moreover, if one knows something, it comes with the responsibility to act on what one knows. And so, it is much easier to posit oneself as a Socrates who "knows nothing" and whose only task is to ask questions, than it is to take a stand for what one knows.

For Descartes, this is what philosophy can become at its worst; an activity in which thought is reduced to nothing else than producing petty questions, fueled by a lack of confidence and a desire for inactivity. Not to think what is, but to flee from it. Not to find what is truly question-worthy, but to avoid facing the real problems plaguing man by wondering away at the most insignificant questions. To question opinion, but only in so far as it separates man from his power and confidence. Crippling one's own natural connection to truth, separating others from their power too, and eventually destroying the possibility of man knowing anything whatsoever, as Epistemon sought to prevent Polyander from thinking. This is pure critique, fueled by the saddest of passions. So long as we are busy questioning what is already perfectly clear, we can postpone the work of creation. So long as we are questioning ourselves, we won't have to build a world. What is philosophy, but the name for all those thoughts that prevent man from thinking? Philosophy says: You are not yet ready to think, and you are not yet ready to believe in your own thought.

When Socrates started philosophizing with the youth of Athens, what did it lead to except a massive decline in confidence? A young man born and bred to be a statesman, feeling in his blood that he already is one, now questioning his own abilities due to the old man Socrates, because upon self-investigation he has realized that he isn't yet fully living in accordance with the Idea of the Statesman. And so, if we do not watch out and let thought, unbound by intuition and common sense, control our entire lives, it can effectively destroy us. For Descartes, as for all great modern philosophers, thought is immensely powerful, and just as it can save us, it can also destroy us.

Descartes' critique of excessive wonder and questioning might seem to contradict a core tenet of his philosophy — hyperbolic doubt. Wasn't he the man who said we should doubt everything? He was, but he said that one should do it at least once in one's life, and certainly not all the time. You would never think of engaging in metaphysical questions during combat. So think, question, and do so in the most radical way possible, but don't doubt if you lack the prerequisite intuition, and don't assume this type of thinking can serve as a guide in each of life's circumstances. In everyday life, we cannot wait for absolute certainty, we have to act on what is probable. And as we have seen, thought has a peculiar way of getting in the way of action.

To guide us in life, we can't just rely on the intellectual intuition needed to grasp metaphysical truths such as "I think, therefore I am." Instead, Descartes mentions a type of bodily intuition or instinct. In daily life, you cannot wait for indubitable certainty before you act on what you know, you have to act on probabilities, guided by instinct, knowing you are doing the best you can with what you know. These instincts find their origin in the body, and it is a characteristic of good health when one can trust one's instincts. We can, for example, imagine a paranoid schizophrenic with all sorts of instincts telling him to do various things, but they are all illusions, and none of them help him.

In this sense, Descartes says that disease or bad health is like an error of nature, for one thing because it literally leads us into error. An organism under stress is more likely to make self-destructive decisions. And so, the instincts of a disturbed body can not be trusted.

It is not that the body is a reservoir of evil inclinations and lies, as some religious fanatics would claim. Rather,

"JUST LIKE OVERTRAINING CAN IMPAIR THE QUALITY OF ONE'S TRAINING, SO OVERTHINKING CAN IMPAIR THE QUALITY OF ONE'S THINKING"

Descartes sees that, depending on its degree of health, the body can either empower us, or destroy us. The same goes for thought: it can empower us, or it can destroy us.

VII. Metabolism and thought

What is health for Descartes? In most simple terms; a state of the body in which everything flows with ease, outside stressors are easily broken down and assimilated, food is easily digested, and nerves easily and accurately transport information to the brain where the soul can get an accurate picture of what is happening to the body. In this process, the heart, referred to as a "fire without light", plays a major role. The heart regulates metabolism, and the stronger the fire burns, the warmer the body, and the faster and easier stressors can be metabolized. The weaker the fire, the more clogged up the body gets.

In the brain, there is the pineal gland, which Descartes speculates to be the seat of the soul. When your hand touches something extremely hot for example, your nerves register this and send a signal to the brain, the information is translated to the soul in the pineal gland, and you get the sensation of hotness. From here, in an almost automatic way, the muscles are activated to move your hand away from the hot object.

This is the basic model for good health — effortless transportation of information, the body being capable of easily metabolizing whatever outside stressor it might encounter, and easily and correctly reacting without having to put in too much effort. This will also be Descartes' ideal of man in general: to be able to make good use of what happens to you, whatever the circumstances. In his principal ethical work, *The Passions of the Soul*, the ethical ideal is not so much to resist the passions in a Stoic manner or to rise above them like an enlightened sage. No, the passions are what make life beautiful, and the best men are not those who don't feel anything, but those who can feel all that life has to offer most intensely, but without letting it drag them down. The noble man can feel the strongest hatred, but he can let it course through him, quickly "metabolize" it, and move on with his life, without letting the hatred fester and grow into a crippling resentment. The noble man does not desire to escape from life, he does not stand above it, he moves through it with grace.

When stressors become too much, either through sheer overload or through the organism being too weak to process them, disease follows. The best course of action? Take some rest, recover your powers, build up energy, and be more sensible in what you take on in the future. It is important to know that these stressors need not be of a physical nature: they can also be thoughts.

As was the case with the excessive wonder of certain philosophical types, or as is the case with too much study or thought acting as a stressor. We all know the experience of feeling drained and empty-headed after a long day of being engaged in intellectual matters. What is peculiar about Descartes is that he integrates this lived experience into his philosophy. Life is not what you do when you cease your philosophical reading or writing, it is not what you do when you leave the university halls. Life is the ground from which you think, and it is what co-determines the power of your thought. And even the most abstract metaphysical projects cannot be undertaken in earnest if not on the basis of a well-ordered life.

And so Descartes is justified in saying that not everyone should undertake his method of universal doubt. Some are just too weak-minded, and questioning everything into oblivion, they will be left with nothing at all. If your thinking is weak, you won't find a certain "I think" at the end of universal doubt. No, your thought will have broken down along the way. Who is it that questions the coherence and certainty of thought? He who is burdened by all sorts of stressors, making his thought and life incapable of the coherence and power needed to stand on their own.

So what is Descartes' fundamental insight? Whether one achieves truth does not depend on the amount of knowledge one has or the number of books one has read. It depends solely on the force of one's thought and on one's confidence, qualities which are as related to the health of one's body as they are related to learning. Dualism: you cannot treat reality from one angle only. If you only 'think', you will no longer be capable of thought.

Just like overtraining can impair the quality of one's training, so overthinking can impair the quality of one's thinking. If you do not take some rest from training, chances are you just dig a hole in your recovery, dragging you further and further away from the gains you seek. The philosophically minded bodybuilder Mike Mentzer understood this well. The same is true with philosophy: Descartes says it is good to take some time off, or you will not get closer to the truth by thinking, but will think yourself further away from it. When you are burdened with stress, intuition —that clarity of thought that allows you to see with the natural light of your reason— it *will* be affected. How will you find the calm needed to contemplate the nature of the soul, when the body is crying out to you for help?

VIII. The decline of intuition: a question of health

In Descartes' famous correspondence with Princess Elisabeth of Bohemia, the princess says she is feeling terribly confused by all the questions they have been pondering about the relation between soul and body, how they are separate substances, yet mysteriously united at the same time. It seems as if, embarking on this search for truth that is philosophy, one only ends up in darkness. Descartes explains that it is very true that, if we do not watch out and conduct our thoughts in an orderly way, philosophy turns from a search for truth into a dwelling in darkness. And, for the really lost, the love of wisdom turns into a love of darkness and obscurity. And so it is of the utmost importance to prevent this 'turning' in which

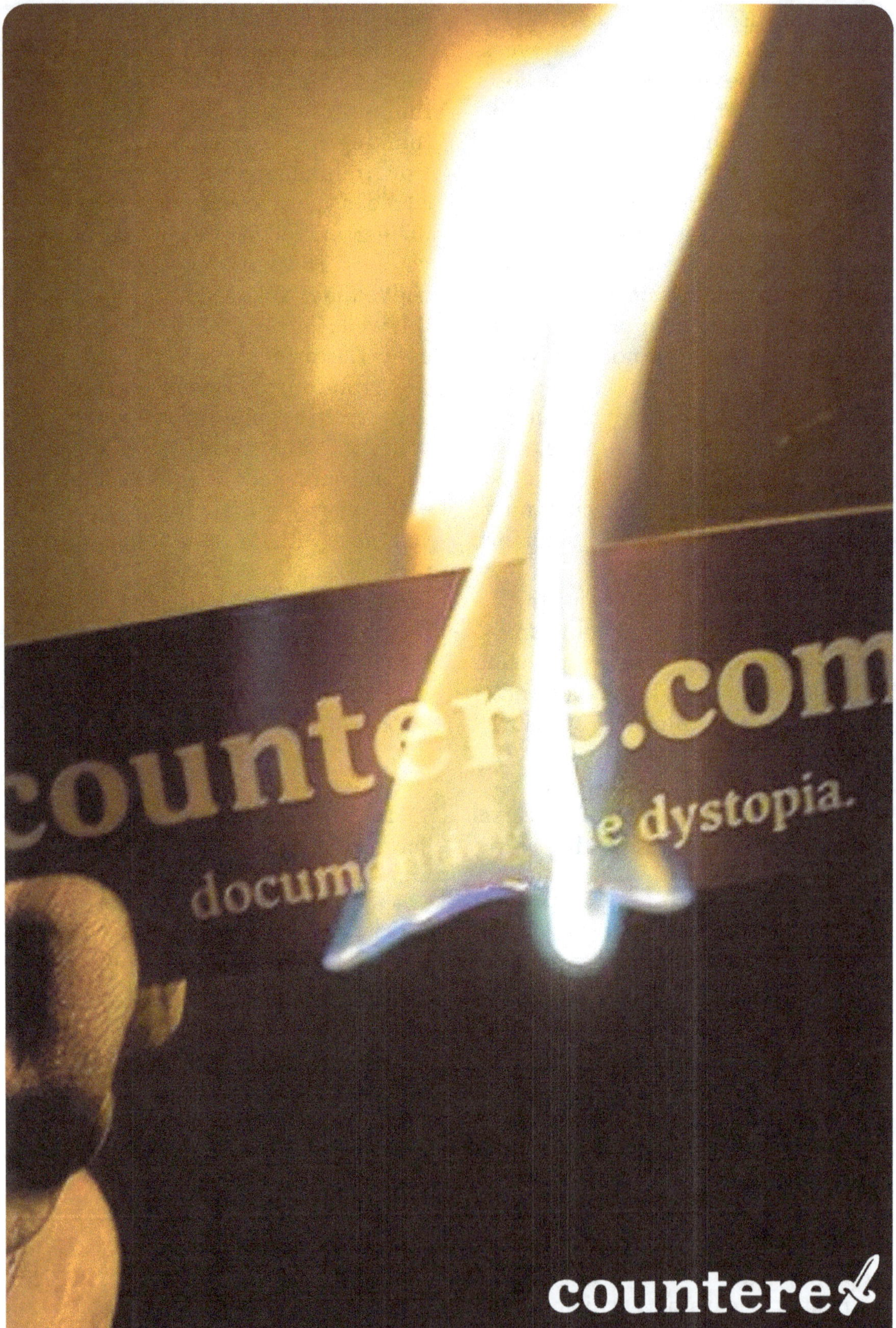

countere.com

document the dystopia.

countere

thought turns against itself.

Descartes goes on to explain how there are three primitive notions — soul, body, and the union of both— each of which is known through a different type of activity:

"Metaphysical thoughts, which exercise the pure intellect, serve to familiarize us with the notion of the soul; and the study of mathematics, which exercises principally the imagination in considering figure and movement, accustoms us to form distinct notions of body. But it is ordinary life and conversation, and the abstention from meditation and the study of things which exercise the imagination, that teaches us how to conceive the union of soul and body."

Descartes says he has always made it a rule to maintain a balance between these three orders in his own life. He tells us it is best to only spend a few hours a day exercising the imagination that leads to clear knowledge of body, and to spend most of the time on "the relaxation of the senses and the repose of the mind." As for the pure metaphysical thinking that detaches itself from the body and leads to familiarity with the soul? "A few hours a year."

If you want to know all there is to know, and maintain sanity, go for a walk. It is a similar theme we will find in Nietzsche — the scholar's terrible expenditure of nervous energy, and the remedy of sun and mountain air.

It is important to know when to use what type of thinking, and there is stupidity in applying the wrong way of thinking to the wrong situation. When doing mathematics, you would be an idiot to let the senses and your bodily instincts interfere with your thinking. Alternatively, only the lowest of thinkers believe that scientific thought can be applied to every area of life. As an example, Descartes mentions those doctors who always think they know better than their patients on the basis of their superior scientific knowledge of the body. But, says Descartes, often the patient's instincts are a more reliable guide to healing than the doctor's knowledge. For the instincts, belonging to the union of soul and body, are Nature speaking directly to the patient. Of course, one can be so totally fucked that one's instincts can no longer be trusted, in which case it is probably better to 'follow the science.' And so it all depends; who is thinking, when, in what way, and why? But here the question arises; who is it that needs logic to guide every moment of his life and thought? What type of man can no longer trust his own instincts and intuition?

Descartes is a philosopher of balance. If pure metaphysical thinking is not balanced with imaginative thinking and relaxation, pure thought itself suffers. When the organism is not in good health, thought ceases being accompanied by intuition, and a mad questioning ensues that is no longer even capable of recognizing truth when it stands before it.

This is Descartes' lesson; think, doubt, and do so in the most radical way possible, but only on the basis of a healthy union of soul and body. Think, radically, but cultivate the intuition to know when your questions are strengthening life, and when they are weakening it. ◼

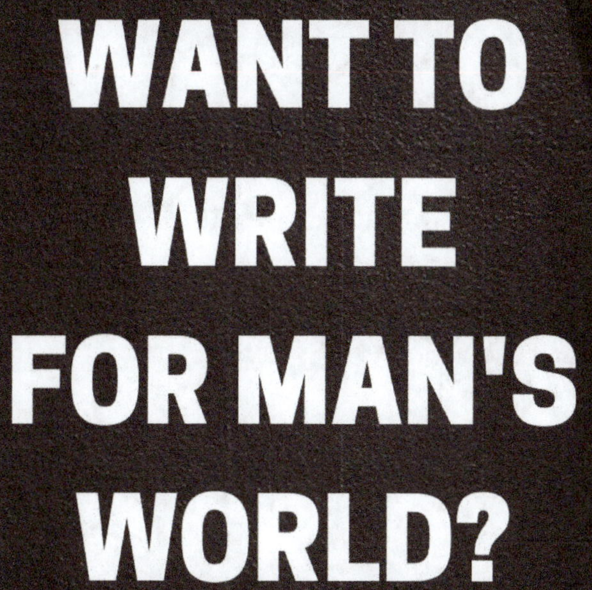

WANT TO WRITE FOR MAN'S WORLD?

If you think you've got something to say,
email mansworldmagazine@protonmail.com